Infertility Solutions

NATURAL APPROACHES

Shana Albo

AVERY

a member of PENGUIN PUTNAM INC.   New York

The information contained in this book is based upon the research and personal and professional experiences of the author. It is not intended as a substitute for consulting with your physician or other health care provider. Any attempt to diagnose and treat an illness or condition should be done under the direction of a health care professional.

The publisher and author are not responsible for any adverse effects or consequences resulting from the use of any of the suggestions, preparations, or procedures discussed in this book. Should the reader have any questions concerning the appropriateness of any procedure or preparation method, the author and the publisher strongly suggest consulting a professional health care advisor.

Most Avery books are available at special quantity discounts for bulk purchase for sales promotions, premiums, fund-raising, and educational needs. Special books or book excerpts also can be created to fit specific needs. For details, write Putnam Special Markets, 375 Hudson Street, New York, NY 10014.

Avery
a member of
Penguin Putnam Inc.
375 Hudson Street
New York, NY 10014
www.penguinputnam.com

Library of Congress Cataloging-in-Publication Data

Albo, Shana.
    Infertility solutions : natural approaches / Shana Albo.
    p. cm.
    Includes bibliographical references and index.
    ISBN: 0-89529-919-4
    1. Infertility. 2. Pregnancy—Complications. I. Title.
    RC889 .A43 2000
    616.6'9206—dc21
                                                    99–35378
                                                    CIP
Printed in the United States of America

10   9   8   7   6   5   4   3   2   1

This book is printed on acid-free paper. ∞

Cover Designer: Phaedra Mastrocola
Typesetter: Gary A. Rosenberg
In-House Editor: Marie Caratozzolo

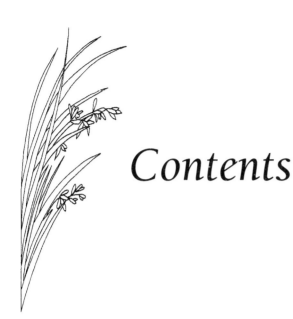

Contents

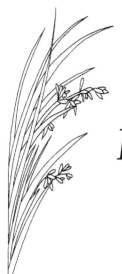

Introduction

*The cure of the part should not be attempted
without treatment of the whole.
No attempt should be made to cure the body
without the soul.*

—Plato

Reproduction, for most human beings, is a relatively easy, natural process requiring limited preparation or forethought. In fact, it is because of this relative ease that 25 percent of all couples who try to get pregnant conceive within the first month, and 85 percent succeed within one year. For the remaining 15 percent of the population, however, fertility is more elusive. It is for this group of people that this book has been written.

My main intention in writing *Infertility Solutions* is to empower couples who are experiencing the pain and heartache of infertility by providing them with a knowledge of holistic alternatives to modern reproductive medicine. Having personally experienced trouble conceiving, I visited a fertility specialist who ran a number of tests to check my ovulatory cycles. In so doing, he determined that my body wasn't releasing the correct levels of hormones and that I wasn't ovulating monthly. The doctor prescribed Clomiphene to "straighten out" my cycles; I took the medication for four months and during this time I became a very "unpleasant" person. The medication caused terrible mood swings and verbally aggressive behavior (what at first I thought was just PMS).

After four months of this ongoing PMS-like behavior and no pregnancy, I decided to stop taking the medication. At that point, I felt that I needed to try a different approach. I had always been interested in alternative (also known as complementary) medicine, and I was determined to explore the area further, not only in the hope of becoming pregnant but also to improve my overall health and to regain the sense of inner balance that I felt I had lost. Fortunately, I found a good physician with a knowledge of alternative treatments. With her help and through my own personal research, I was able to devise a program that strengthened my mind-body state naturally, which increased my odds of conceiving.

The advice provided in this book is the culmination of my research on reproduction. It explains how the environment, improper nutrition, and stress, among other things, can affect the reproductive system. As you progress from chapter to chapter, you will gain knowledge of a number of effective complementary therapies that help you to incorporate those aspects most suitable for you. As I will reiterate often, no one treatment is a panacea for everyone. Treatment is as individual as the patient.

The human body exists as a whole. As such, it is important that each individual part feels well in order for the other parts to function properly. Our "whole" self is intertwined with the environment that surrounds us. We can't feel well if we live in polluted or otherwise unhealthy surroundings, or if we find ourselves filled with stress, anxiety, or tension. We absorb our surroundings, and our bodies reflect this. To maintain a healthy mind-body state, we must live in an environment that promotes health and well-being. While researching the material for this book, I became increasingly aware of how important this is. Moreover, if we do not live in such a nurturing environment, our well-being—that of our mind, body, and spirit—certainly will be compromised.

The suggestions offered in the following chapters are meant to enhance your health, your lifestyle, and your entire mind-body state in order to encourage fertility. The challenge may at first seem daunting, if not overwhelming, but it is possible. Sometimes, all that is required is a change of diet or the elimination of the use of cigarettes or alcohol. Whatever path you choose, be assured that it will not just improve your chances of becoming pregnant, it will also help you look at yourself and your environment in a healthier, more holistic way.

1

Reproduction

This chapter presents the intricacies of the female and male reproductive systems. Before discussing the various causes of infertility and some of its effective, natural treatment methods, it is important to first understand the basic reproductive process.

FEMALE REPRODUCTIVE SYSTEM

The female reproductive system, as illustrated in Figure 1.1, includes the ovaries, fallopian tubes, uterus, and vagina, as well as the hypothalamus and the pituitary glands. With the exception of the hypothalamus and pituitary glands, which are located in the brain, these organs are found in the pelvic area.

The *uterus*, also known as the *womb*, is the principal organ involved in pregnancy. Similar in shape to an upside down pear, the uterus houses the growing fetus. The entrance to the uterus is known as the *cervix*. Two *ovaries*, each about the size of an almond, are located on either side of the uterus. The

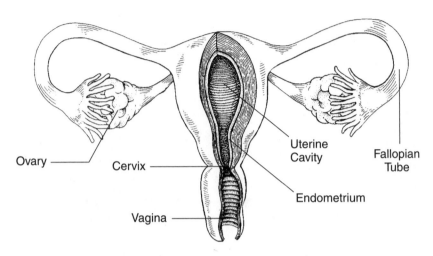

Figure 1.1. Female Reproductive System

ovaries have two main functions—they house eggs or *ova,* and they produce the hormones *estrogen* and *progesterone.* These hormones are responsible for the menstrual cycle and female characteristics such as breast development. They are also important for the development of the fetus after fertilization. Two slender, hollow ducts called *fallopian tubes* curve out from the uterus and end in small projections that surround the ovaries. The fallopian tubes transport the eggs from the ovaries to the uterus. The *vagina* is the passage that extends from the cervix to the external genitals.

The Menstrual Cycle

Beginning with the time a female reaches puberty and has her first menstrual period, her reproductive system controls her monthly menstrual cycle. The average menstrual cycle lasts about twenty-eight days, but often varies from twenty-five to thirty-five days. The menstrual cycle consists of three phases—follicular, ovulatory, and luteal. These phases are detailed in the following discussion and summarized in Table 1.1 on page 9.

The Follicular Phase

The female menstrual cycle begins with the follicular phase during which follicles develop. During this phase, *estradiol* (an estrogen) and *progesterone* levels are low. This triggers the uterus to shed its lining, resulting in *menstruation*. (If a released egg had been fertilized during the previous cycle, this endometrial lining would have nourished the growing embryo.) Bleeding signifies the first day of the woman's menstrual cycle. While estrogen and progesterone remain low during menstruation, the *hypothalamus* (a small gland in the brain) produces *gonadotropic hormone* (GnRH). High levels of GnRH stimulate the *pituitary gland* to release *follicle-stimulating hormone* (FSH) and *luteinizing hormone* (LH). Slightly increased levels of FSH encourage the development of several follicles, each ideally containing an egg. Typically, only one of these follicles continues to develop.

The Ovulatory Phase

Generally, by the thirteenth or fourteenth days of an average twenty-eight day menstrual cycle, the pituitary gland produces a surge in luteinizing and follicle-stimulating hormones. This marks the end of the follicular phase and the beginning of the ovulatory phase. At this point, LH levels have reached their peak, and the egg follicle is ready to be

So Many Eggs

Unlike sperm, which are produced constantly, all of the eggs a female will ever have—about 2 million—are present in her ovaries at birth. No more develop. By the time menstruation begins, anywhere from 40,000 to 300,000 immature eggs remain. And only a few hundred will ever reach maturity and be released—usually one during each menstrual cycle—during a woman's reproductive years.

released from the ovary. Ovulation occurs when the fully mature follicle releases its egg, as seen in Figure 1.2. This usually occurs from sixteen to thirty-two hours after the LH surge begins. The exact day of ovulation may vary from month to month, but it is always triggered by a surge in LH hormone levels. During the surge, estradiol levels peak and progesterone begins to increase. Once released, the egg can live for twelve to twenty-four hours. (The longevity of the egg is an important factor in timing intercourse right before ovulation.)

The Luteal Phase

The luteal phase follows ovulation and, unless fertilization occurs, lasts about fourteen days. It ends just before the next menstrual cycle begins. During this phase, levels of luteinizing hormone and follicle-stimulating hormone decrease. The ruptured follicle closes after releasing the egg and forms the *corpus luteum*, as shown in Figure 1.2. Situated on the surface of the ovary, the corpus luteum is 1 to 2 centimeters in diameter and responsible for secreting progesterone. Along with estradiol, progesterone causes the uterine lining (the endometrium) to thicken in preparation for a fertilized egg. If fertilization does not occur, the corpus luteum degenerates, resulting in menstruation. If, however, an egg is fertilized, the

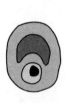 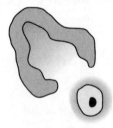

The follicle
matures during the follicular phase . . .   *releases an egg during the ovulatory phase . . .*   *and develops into the corpus luteum during the luteal phase.*

Figure 1.2. Follicle Maturation

Table 1.1. Menstrual Cycle Phases

Follicular Phase Days 1–12	Ovulatory Phase Days 13–15	Luteal Phase Days 16–28
• Endometrial lining sheds, marking the beginning of the cycle. • Follicle-stimulating hormone levels increase, stimulating new follicle development.	• Begins with surge of luteinizing hormone. • Mature follicle releases egg.	• Luteinizing and follicle-stimulating hormones decrease. • Follicle develops into the corpus luteum. • Progesterone and estradiol cause thickening of uterine lining (endometrium). • If conception doesn't occur, the uterine lining sheds, marking the beginning of a new cycle.

* The information above is based on an average twenty-eight-day cycle. Phase lengths are approximate.

corpus luteum will continue to produce progesterone until the fetus can produce its own.

MALE REPRODUCTIVE SYSTEM

As seen in Figure 1.3, the external structures of the male reproductive system are the penis, scrotum, and testes (testicles). The vas deferens, urethra, prostate gland, and seminal vesicles are the internal structures. The male's genes are carried within *sperm*, which is produced in the testes and stored in the seminal vesicles.

Attached to the abdominal wall, the *penis* consists of a root, body, and cone-shaped head called the *glans penis*. The

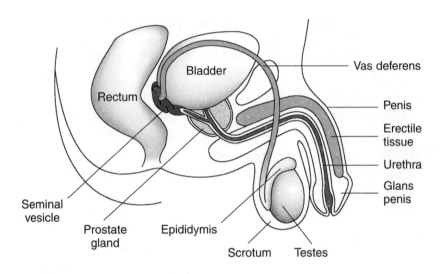

Figure 1.3. Male Reproductive System

urethra is the channel that transports both semen and urine; its opening is located at the tip of the glans penis.

A thin-skinned sac called the *scrotum* surrounds the *testes,* which are small oval-shaped structures that produce sperm and synthesize *testosterone*—the primary male sex hormone. In order for normal sperm to develop, the testes must be cooler than the rest of the body. The scrotum allows the testes to hang away from the body to help maintain the appropriate temperature. Lying against the testes is the *epididymis*—a long coiled tube that collects the sperm. It is here that the sperm matures. This maturation period takes approximately three months.

The *vas deferens* is a duct that transports sperm from the epididymis. It travels along the back of the prostate gland to the urethra, where it forms ejaculatory ducts. Surrounding part of the urethra, the *prostate gland* lies under the bladder. Along with the *seminal vesicles,* the prostate gland produces the greatest volume of *semen,* the fluid that transports the sperm.

When stimulated, the penis becomes rigid, enabling vaginal penetration during sexual intercourse. During ejaculation, nerves stimulate muscle contractions along the ducts of the vas deferens, the seminal vesicles, and the prostate. These contractions force semen into the urethra, which also contracts, further expelling semen through and out of the penis.

Once in the female genital tract, sperm have a relatively short life span. While their capability for swimming may last up to three or four days, their fertilizing ability usually lasts only twenty-four hours. And although a typical ejaculation deposits millions of sperm in the vagina, generally, only a few thousand reach the site of fertilization in the fallopian tube.

DETERMINING OVULATION

When trying to conceive, determining the time of ovulation is very important, although not necessarily an easy task. As explained earlier, typically, human ova live in the female reproductive tract for only twenty-four hours. In addition, the fertile period of time in the *average* twenty-eight-day menstrual cycle falls somewhere between days twelve and fourteen. Generally, fertility peaks on approximately the fourteenth day of this cycle. (Keep in mind that most women experience menstrual cycles that vary in length from month to month, and ovulation does not necessarily occur on day fourteen of every cycle.) For an increased chance of conception, intercourse should, therefore, take place from four days prior to the suspected time of ovulation to a couple of days after ovulation has occurred. Some experts do not recommend frequent intercourse during this time period as the strength and motility of the sperm may be weakened.

Determining the time of ovulation can be tricky. Charting basal body temperature and analyzing cervical mucus are two techniques for helping to determine this time.

Cycle Day	1	2	3	4	5	6	7	8	9	10	11	12	13
Date													
99.2°F													
99.0°F													
98.8°F													
98.6°F													
98.4°F													
98.2°F													
98.0°F													
97.8°F													
97.6°F													
97.4°F													
97.2°F													
97.0°F													
96.8°F													
96.6°F													
96.4°F													

Basal Body Temperature Chart

Charting Basal Body Temperature

Charting one's basal body temperature—a technique that has been used for many years—can be effective in determining the time of ovulation. Generally, a woman's body temperature ranges from 97°F to 98.6°F. A drop of one-half to one full degree in this average temperature usually occurs just before a significant rise in temperature—an indication that ovulation is about to occur. The ideal time to have intercourse is when the temperature begins to climb to its highest rise. If there is

14	15	16	17	18	19	20	21	22	23	24	25	26	27	28

little body temperature change throughout the cycle, chances are ovulation did not occur.

When using the basal body method to determine the time of ovulation, simply take your temperature before rising out of bed in the morning. Using the chart above, record your findings. When you see your temperature drop then rise sharply, chances are you are beginning to ovulate. Monitor your temperature for a few cycles. Also, be sure to make note of any unusual circumstances, such as days on which you might be ill, fatigued from a poor night's sleep, or unusually stressed.

It is also recommended that you use a special basal temperature thermometer—not a regular oral or digital type. Basal thermometers, which are available in most pharmacies, are more sensitive to minute changes in body temperature than other types.

Analyzing Cervical Mucus

Using the basal body temperature method of determining time of ovulation can be made even more effective by combining it with the cervical mucus method. Analyzing cervical mucus as a method of determining time of ovulation was developed by Doctors John and Evelyn Billings. Many women use this method both as a means of conceiving, as well as avoiding pregnancy.

Simply observing changes in cervical mucus can help determine fertile periods during the menstrual cycle. Prior to ovulation, the mucus is very cloudy, acidic, and thick, preventing sperm from entering the uterus. As ovulation nears, the mucus becomes more stretchy and alkaline in nature. During ovulation, high estrogen levels cause the mucus to become very liquidy and clear, naturally encouraging sperm to enter the uterus.

Using an Ovulation Predictor Kit

At-home easy-to-use test kits for predicting ovulation are available in most pharmacies. These fairly accurate tests detect increased levels of luteinizing hormone in the urine. As you have learned, increased levels of this hormone signify ovulation.

THE AGE FACTOR

Age is another factor in ensuring optimum fertility. Fertility rates peak when a woman is in her early and mid-twenties, and decrease as she gets older. After age thirty-eight, a woman is 30 percent less fertile than a woman in her twenties. Although ideally, women should conceive in their twenties, economic and social conditions do not always make this a feasible option. Since the late 1980s, the number of women having their first child after age thirty-five has skyrocketed in North America. Increasing numbers of women are putting off getting married and building a family until they feel financially secure. By this time, however, the female biological clock is often starting to wind down, and becoming pregnant may be more challenging.

SUMMING IT UP

There you have it—the basics of reproduction and some effective ways of determining time of ovulation. Now it's time to move on to the next chapter, which presents a number of common causes of infertility.

2

Causes of Infertility

Infertility is commonly defined as the inability to conceive after approximately twelve months of sexual activity without the use of birth control. Since fertility naturally declines with age, women thirty-five years of age and older should consult a fertility specialist if they have not conceived after six months.

Approximately 15 percent of all couples, literally millions of Americans, experience difficulty with conception. Major physiological causes of infertility include problems with sperm, the uterus, the fallopian tubes, the ovaries, the cervix, and the corpus luteum, as well as hormone imbalances. Many forms of infertility are the result of actual damage to the reproductive system, either through disease or infection, and may require medical or technological attention. In quite a few cases, however, abnormalities of the sperm, the cervical mucus, and the corpus luteum, as well as hormone imbalances have been shown to react positively to natural alternative treatments. For instance, combining a nutrient-rich diet with certain herbs, stress-reduction techniques, and therapies such as aromatherapy and acupuncture, has been shown to have positive effects in increasing fertility.

Exposure to environmental pollutants, as well as poor lifestyle choices, such as smoking, drinking alcohol, eating nutrient-deficient diets, and living with constant stress, can seriously impair fertility in both men and women. In fact, numerous studies have linked chemicals and environmental toxins, as well as stress and poor nutrition to hormone imbalances in women. Unfortunately, traditional medicine often tends to ignore these factors when treating infertility.

PROBLEMS WITH SPERM

In the adult male, sperm formation in the testes is continuous. To be considered fertile, a male must be able to deliver an adequate quantity of normal sperm to the female. The average volume of semen per ejaculation is 4 milliliters, containing as many as 350 million sperm. Of these, a minimum of 80 million motile sperm is considered necessary for fertility. Typically, a variety of sperm types is found in each ejaculate, of which only one type is considered normal. An inadequate sperm count and poorly structured sperm are responsible for infertility in a substantial percentage of couples. Poor sperm motility is another common cause.

As discussed in Chapter 1, sperm formation is most efficient at a temperature of about 93°F, which is lower than the normal body temperature. Because the testes—where sperm are formed—are located outside the body cavity in the scrotum, they can be kept at this lower temperature.

A *varicocele*—a mass of varicose-type veins in the scrotum—is the most common physical cause of infertility in men. It may prevent proper blood drainage from the testes, raising their temperature and reducing the rate of sperm formation. In some cases, varicoceles can be treated successfully with minor surgery.

Inadequate sperm production and poor motility may also

be caused by prolonged exposure to heat from hot showers, baths, saunas, or steam baths; from wearing tight-fitting underwear, athletic supporters, jeans, or slacks; or from using electric blankets. Other causes include exposure to environmental toxins, including radiation, heavy metals, and air pollutants. Cigarette smoking and the use of street drugs such as marijuana are other culprits.

UTERINE ABNORMALITIES

The pear-shaped uterus consists of three layers of tissue—the *parametrium,* the *myometrium,* and the *endometrium.* It is the endometrium that undergoes the continual forming and shedding during the monthly menstrual cycle. In the case of conception, the uterus provides a home in which the embryo implants itself.

Some cases of infertility are the result of *pelvic inflammato-*

The Effects of DES

DES (diethylstilbestrol)—a synthetic estrogen derived from coal tar—was commonly prescribed for pregnant women from the 1940s to the early 1970s to prevent miscarriage. What was unforeseen at that time, however, was the downside of DES. According to the "Journal of the American Medical Association," many offspring of the more than 3 million women in the United States who took DES developed serious reproductive problems. Damage to females included uterine abnormalities; incompetent cervixes, which resulted in difficulty in carrying a pregnancy to term; and increased risks of infertility, fibroid tumors, and uterine cancer. A number of male offspring experienced a blockage of the vas deferens, leading to sterility.

ry disease (PID), caused by the sexually transmitted diseases chlamydia and gonorrhea. Pelvic inflammatory disease—an infection of the reproductive tract—is commonly characterized by symptoms that include burning upon urination, bladder discomfort, pelvic pain, and abnormal bleeding between menstrual periods. In many women, however, chlamydia and gonorrhea are asymptomatic—they cause no symptoms. In such cases, these diseases go untreated until inflammation sets in. In most cases, especially when treated early enough, uterine infections can be cured with antibiotics. Untreated, PID leads to infertility in approximately one out of ten infected women.

A malformed or misshapen uterus and/or blocked fallopian tubes can cause problems with conception. Congenital birth defects, fibroid tumors, and scar tissue from pelvic infections can make embryo implantation difficult. Endometriosis, discussed below, is another possible cause. Scarring outside the fallopian tubes can prevent an egg from entering or passing through, while scarring within the uterus can prevent a fertilized egg from becoming implanted in the uterine lining. These conditions also can cause miscarriages early in pregnancy. A *hysterosalpingogram*—an x-ray that is taken after dye is injected into the uterus and fallopian tubes—can determine if there is a malformation of the uterus or a blockage of the fallopian tubes. Both of these conditions are serious and require conventional medical intervention (namely surgery or the use of modern reproductive technology).

Endometriosis is a disease that affects 10 million American women of childbearing age. In it, cells that form the endometrium, which normally grow inside the uterus where they support the development of a fertilized egg, also grow outside the uterus. These endometrial tissue growths, also called *implants,* occur in or around the ovaries, the fallopian tubes, the urinary bladder, and the pelvic floor. In some cases, the cell tissue also spreads to areas outside the reproductive system, such as the abdominal cavity.

Although they are not located within the uterus, these abnormal implants respond to the changes in progesterone and estrogen levels that control menstruation. Like the uterine lining, these growths build tissue each month, then break down and bleed. Unlike blood from the uterine lining, however, blood from endometrial implants has no way to leave the body, and must, instead, be absorbed by surrounding tissue. This absorption process takes a long time, and blood often accumulates. Month after month, these implants get larger and larger and may form blood-filled cysts and scar tissue. In severe cases, the scarring and adhesions interfere with ovulation, fertilization, and embryo implantation.

Common symptoms of endometriosis include intense pain in the pelvic area prior to and during menstruation; sporadic pain throughout the menstrual cycle; painful intercourse; excessive bleeding, including the passing of large clots during menstruation; and nausea, vomiting, and constipation during menstruation.

Endometriosis is sometimes misdiagnosed by physicians who mistake it for ovarian cysts, pelvic inflammatory disease, or premenstrual syndrome. For this reason, women experiencing any of the above-mentioned symptoms who are also experiencing problems with fertility should see a physician.

Laser laparoscopy is used to diagnose endometriosis. During this procedure, a tiny optical tube with a light is inserted into the abdominal cavity through a small incision in the navel. The surgeon is then able to look inside the abdominal cavity for endometrial tissue growing outside the uterus.

Traditional treatments for endometriosis and the infertility that may result are based on trying to stop the spread of the disease and repair the damage that already has occurred. Treatments include laser laparoscopy in which endometrial tissue outside the reproductive system is removed. Clomiphene, an anti-estrogen fertility drug (normally used to stimulate ovulation in women) is sometimes prescribed to help treat endometriosis.

A nutrient program consisting of foods high in vitamins B, C, and E, and selenium may help alleviate endometriosis. Because high levels of estrogen are needed to build endometrial tissue, removing excess estrogen from the body is helpful in easing endometriosis. According to Dr. Susan M. Lark, author of *Fibroid Tumors and Endometriosis: A Self-Help Book,* the B vitamins help the liver break down and eliminate excess estrogen from the body. Vitamins C and E, and selenium, are powerful antioxidants that can help ease menstrual cramps and reduce heavy bleeding.

Women suffering from endometriosis should also reduce their intake of caffeine and dairy-products. Dairy products contain saturated fats, which put a strain on the liver and increase the circulating estrogen in the body. (High levels of estrogen may exacerbate the problem of endometriosis by causing endometrial tissue to build up outside the uterus.) For this same reason, it is recommended that women with endometriosis also reduce caffeine intake—caffeine slows down proper liver function, which may increase estrogen levels in the body.

TUBAL ABNORMALITIES

As explained in Chapter 1, the fallopian tubes are a pair of ducts located on both sides of the uterus that lead to the ovaries. Each month, ideally, one or both ovaries releases an egg, which is then swept into the fallopian tube where it makes its way to the uterus. During this journey, if the egg comes into contact with sperm, conception and implantation in the uterus should occur. Some women, however, have a blockage or scarring in their fallopian tubes, making conception difficult or impossible. Common causes of tubal abnormalities include:

- Endometriosis.

- Cysts (fluid-filled sacs).

- A sexually transmitted disease such as chlamydia or gonorrhea.

- Scarring from the use of an intrauterine birth control device (IUD).

- Inflammation within the reproductive tract, often the result of an infection.

When the fallopian tubes become blocked, scarred, or otherwise damaged due to infection or inflammation, the egg and sperm are unable to pass freely through the tubes, and conception can be difficult, if not impossible. An antibiotic may be able to clear up a bacterial infection such as chlamydia or gonorrhea, or a genital mycoplasma infection, without much damage to the reproductive tract. (Chlamydia and gonorrhea are two types of bacteria that are easily contracted through sexual intercourse. Genital mycoplasmas are microbes—neither bacterial nor viral—that are also sexually transmitted, and can be treated with antibiotics.) However, if not treated in time, the fallopian tubes may become very badly scarred or blocked, and surgery or another technological procedure may be necessary to increase the chances of conception. In some cases, conception may occur, but implantation may take place outside the uterus, resulting in an *ectopic pregnancy*—a potentially life-threatening condition that requires immediate medical intervention.

OVARIAN ABNORMALITIES

The ovaries are two small, round glands, approximately three centimeters long and two centimeters wide, that produce ova and the sex hormones estrogen and progesterone. Each month, one or both of the ovaries typically release an egg, which travels through the fallopian tube to the uterus. Infertility due to an ovarian abnormality may be caused by:

- Malformed ovaries.

- Ovarian cysts.

- Adhesions to the lining of the ovaries as a result of inflammation, either from an infection, such as gonorrhea or chlamydia, or as the result of gynecological or abdominal surgery.

- Anovulation (lack of ovulation) due to a hormonal imbalance.

Ultrasound scans and/or a laparoscopy are generally used to diagnose ovarian abnormalities. As ova are clearly visible through ultrasound, a scan can help determine if a woman is ovulating regularly or even at all. An ultrasound scan will also detect ovarian cysts and malformed ovaries. Surgery can help correct ovarian cysts, while fertility drugs, such as Clomiphene and Pergonal, are commonly used to treat anovulation. In some cases of very serious ovarian and tubal abnormalities, reproductive endocrinologists may suggest technological methods such as *in vitro* fertilization (IVF). Through IVF, unfertilized eggs are removed from the ovaries and fertilized with sperm. They are then placed back in the woman's uterus where, hopefully, they will implant.

PROBLEMS OF THE CERVIX

Cervical mucus acts as a filter, preventing vaginal bacteria from entering the uterus. The mucus also plays an important role in aiding sperm survival. Depending on the time of the menstrual cycle, the mucus changes texture, quantity, and color. Prior to ovulation, the mucus is cloudy and thick and impenetrable to sperm. However, when the egg is maturing in the ovary—the follicular phase of the menstrual cycle— increased levels of the hormone estradiol change the mucus to a very clear, stretchy substance. Sperm can move easily through this mucus into the uterus, then to the fallopian tubes.

Thick, cloudy, and/or acidic cervical mucus can be the result of a hormone imbalance, a vaginal infection, or the use of antihistamines. Some women have certain antibodies in their mucus that perceive sperm as foreign invaders and destroy or immobilize them.

In order to diagnose cervical mucus abnormalities, a series of analytical medical tests is required. If these tests determine the woman is producing antibodies to male sperm, antibiotics may be prescribed. For women whose cervical mucus is highly acidic, which neutralizes sperm, a low-acid diet may be recommended. Another alternative for women with cervical mucus problems is artificial insemination. Through this process, sperm bypass the cervical mucus and is introduced into the uterus through mechanical means.

CORPUS LUTEUM ABNORMALITIES

As explained in Chapter 1, the main function of the corpus luteum is to produce progesterone, which is crucial for form-ing and maintaining the endometrial lining of the uterus. If conception occurs, progesterone levels remain high and con-tinue to strengthen the endometrium, which provides a "home" for the fertilized egg as it grows and develops into an embryo. If conception does not occur, the corpus luteum pro-duces less and less progesterone, and it begins to decompose during the final phase of the menstrual cycle until it is little more than a pale spot on the surface of the ovary. Without the necessary progesterone, the endometrial lining sheds, mark-ing the beginning of menstruation.

Women who suffer from abnormalities of the corpus luteum, such as *luteal phase defect,* often ovulate but do not produce high enough levels of progesterone. Without the proper levels of progesterone, the endometrial lining of the uterus is not prepared for the implanted fertilized egg. And

Sperm Under Attack

Some women produce antibodies to their partner's sperm. For some reason, sperm is perceived as a hostile invader and antibodies attack it. Women who produce such antibodies should have their partners wear condoms during intercourse for a few months before trying to conceive. By reducing a woman's exposure to her partner's sperm, her body may get the chance it needs to stop producing these antibodies. When condom-free intercourse occurs, her partner's sperm may have a better chance of reaching and fertilizing her ova.

even if the egg does implant itself, the weak lining won't be able to maintain it. The result is a miscarriage. Women with luteal phase defect typically have very short menstrual cycles.

Luteal phase defect is typically diagnosed by a serum progesterone test or an ultrasound scan. From a blood sample that is taken seven to nine days after ovulation, a *serum progesterone test* is able to determine progesterone production of the corpus luteum. An *ultrasound scan,* also performed seven to nine days after ovulation, can determine if the corpus luteum is producing enough progesterone by analyzing the width of the uterine lining. Doctors have traditionally offered patients progesterone therapy during the second half of their menstrual cycle to treat this form of infertility.

Complementary medicine offers a number of approaches for treating luteal phase defect. Two herbs—dong quai and red raspberry leaves—may be beneficial as they help encourage the body to produce progesterone naturally. Another effective way to help balance the body's progesterone levels is by using natural progesterone cream. Traditionally prescribed for premenopausal women, natural progesterone cream is 100 percent bioavailable and does not put undo strain on the liver. The cream should contain at least 400 milliliters of natural progesterone per ounce. It should be applied to the soft tissue areas of the body such as the stomach and the thighs, from the day of ovulation (often the fourteenth day of a typical twenty-eight day cycle) until the first day of the next menstrual cycle.

HORMONAL IMBALANCE

Hormone imbalances are a common cause of female infertility. This is due primarily to the sensitivity of the endocrine system, which regulates hormone production.

The menstrual cycle is an extremely complicated and timed coordination between the body's hormones, its reproductive organs, and the hypothalamus. Not only must each be functioning properly, but they must do so in a timely and balanced manner. As seen in Chapter 1, five hormones— gonadotropic hormone (GnRH), follicle-stimulating hormone (FSH), luteinizing hormone (LH), estrogen, and progesterone—are present in varying degrees during the menstrual cycle. It is this very delicate balance in rising and falling hormone levels that determines when a woman can become pregnant. Even minor fluctuations in hormone balances can result in irregular or infrequent menstrual periods, a lack of ovulation (anovulation), and infertility.

If the hypothalamus does not produce a sufficient amount of GnRH, the pituitary gland, in turn, cannot produce the important follicle-stimulating hormone and luteinizing hormone. If either of these two hormones is not released, a follicle may not develop; and if a follicle does not mature and release its egg, ovulation cannot occur. If progesterone levels are inadequately low, even if an egg is fertilized, the endometrial lining will not be thick enough to enable the embryo to implant itself in the uterus. Moreover, if proper estrogen levels are not maintained throughout the menstrual cycle, the endometrial lining will not be able to form at all.

Stress, psychological and emotional disturbances, and inadequate nutritional intake all can disrupt hormonal balance in the human body. There is also increasing evidence that "estrogen mimicking" chemicals in our environment are capable of disrupting human hormone levels, causing reproductive problems. (The effects of these chemicals—also known as endocrine disrupters—are discussed at length in Chapter 3). Eventually, these factors accumulate and disrupt the overall internal harmony within the body, creating what conventional medicine defines as a hormonal imbalance. Therefore, if only the symptom (or symptoms) is treated, and the entire body remains blocked physically, emotionally, and spiritually, eventually and inevitably, another symptom will appear.

Traditional medicine typically treats hormone imbalances with fertility drugs such as Clomiphene and Menotropins. Treating this form of infertility with medication alone may rebalance hormone levels, but it ignores the underlying causes. New research indicates that there might be a link between hormone imbalance in the human reproductive system and stress and diet. It is important to both rebalance hormonal levels and heal the entire body. If stress is the cause of infertility, forms of stress management techniques should be practiced (see Chapter 8).

THE GENE CONNECTION

Recent, groundbreaking research in the field of genetics has brought to light a connection between defective genes in the human DNA (the genetic information contained in the chromosomes of the nucleus of living cells) and infertility. About 10 percent of male infertility is due to genetics, according to Dr. Marc Goldstein, director of the Center for Male Reproductive Medicine and microsurgery at the New York Hospital

Cornell Medical Center. Recent research performed on laboratory mice indicate a link between faulty genes (namely the A-MYB gene, the Dhh gene, and the CREM gene) and some types of male infertility. Researchers at Temple University School of Medicine, Fels Institute for Cancer Research, are currently working on gene therapy to help men suffering from genetically-related forms of infertility. Although more studies must be conducted, this latest research on the role of genetics in infertility is very encouraging.

According to current genetic research, women with consistently low levels of luteinizing hormone (LH) may have a faulty NGFI-A gene. This gene regulates the production of LH in women, thereby controlling ovulation. In some women, however, this gene either does not exist or it is defective, preventing ovulation. Typical conventional treatment includes the use of fertility drugs to raise LH levels in the body and stimulate ovulation. Chaste tree (*Vitex agnus-castus*), an herb common to the Mediterranean region, is a nonprescription alternative remedy. This herb was recommended by the Greek physician Hippocrates 2,500 years ago, as a remedy for balancing female hormone levels, specifically luteinizing hormone. Chapter 6 presents more information on herbal treatments.

OTHER INFERTILITY CAUSES

Unexplained infertility may be caused by a vitamin deficiency, poor diet, cigarette smoking, alcohol and caffeine consumption, heavy metal and chemical exposure, and, of course, stress. (All of these factors will be discussed in detail in later chapters.)

According to a research study conducted in 1997 by psychologist Alice Domar, frequent bouts of depression and stress may impair reproductive function and increase the chances of becoming infertile. Dr. Donar conducted a ten-week stress management program at the Beth Israel

Deaconess Medical Center in Boston, for 174 women suffering from infertility problems and various levels of depression. Each woman had been trying to become pregnant for an average of three years, and all were suffering from clinical depression. Within six months of completing the program, 60 percent of the women who had originally scored the highest on depression tests, became pregnant. Among the least depressed, 25 percent conceived within six months of completing the program. Dr. Donar concluded that improving the mood of extremely depressed, infertile women might induce hormone shifts that contribute to ovulation.

Typically, physicians tend to pay a lot of attention to treating infertile patients through surgery, drugs, and modern reproductive technology, while paying minimal attention to the environmental, psychological, and biological culprits that may be at the root of the problem. And some patients who are desperate for a child after years of infertility will take any medication or undergo any treatment available for the chance to become pregnant.

While modern reproductive technology is certainly miraculous and has been a godsend for thousands of infertile couples, it is not a panacea for all. In addition to the high cost factor associated with fertility drugs and other special treatments, their success rates vary. In vitro fertilization (IVF), for example, has a success rate of 22 percent (although some clinics claim a higher success rate). Fertility drugs have a much higher success rate; however, they may also increase the chance of multiple births and may predispose a woman to ovarian cancer later in life. According to a study conducted by Dr. Mary Avner Rossing and coworkers at the University of Washington and Fred Hutchinson Cancer Research Center, women treated with infertility drugs have a 2.5 times higher risk of ovarian cancer than the general population. These results were based on a study of 3,837 women between 1974 and 1986 in the Seattle area. Earlier research conducted by scientists from the United States also indicate a possible correlation between certain infertility treatments and ovarian cancer.

For some women, there are no obvious physiological causes of infertility. They have a well-functioning reproductive system, yet they still are unable to become pregnant. In such cases, these women may have what Julian and Susan Scott describe in their book *Natural Medicine for Women* as a "weak energy pattern . . . a lack of energy in the reproductive system. This lack of vitality in the uterus—although not obvious from medical tests—is unable to quicken life. This may be due to an overall lack of energy when [they] feel tired, or to a specific lack of energy in the reproductive system . . ."

The concept of human energy flow and disease is not readily accepted by Western medicine, and is equally difficult to prove scientifically. However, in the Far East, it is believed that energy (chi) flows through the human body. In fact, shiatsu, acupuncture, and reflexology—three methods of healing that originated in Asia—are based on the concept of human energy (chi) and its ability to flow through the body. When a person is emotionally healthy and relaxed, the energy in his or her body flows vigorously, enabling it to function well. However, when a person is under stress or is tired, he or she may not have enough strength to channel that energy. This may lead to "energy blockage," which can eventually cause long-term disease symptoms in the area of the body that is "blocked."

In the Far East, a blockage of energy in the reproductive system area of the body is believed to be a valid cause for infertility in some women. This type of infertility is often not diagnosed by Western doctors because it does not show any outward symptoms that can be analyzed by medical tests. Nonetheless, women who are under emotional distress or who feel tired or stressed regularly may find popular Eastern methods of healing, such as acupressure, reflexology, or massage, beneficial. Chapter 8 presents these stress-reducing techniques in detail.

SUMMING IT UP

Infertility resulting from inadequate or poorly structured sperm, or a tubal, ovarian, or uterine abnormality may be helped by surgery or other modern reproductive methods. However, if you are having difficulty becoming pregnant and do not have an abnormality or infection within the reproductive system, then such factors as stress, vitamin deficiency, and environmental toxins may be at the root of your problem. In such cases, stress-management techniques, relaxation, and proper nutrition may help rebalance and strengthen your reproductive system, as well as your mind and body.

3

Environment and Lifestyle

As male sperm counts plummet worldwide, and as female infertility is now linked, at least in part, to such lifestyle choices as smoking, alcohol consumption, poor diet, lack of exercise, and use of medications, everyone has reason to be concerned. The problem is not getting better. And it is only within the last few years that Western governments and scientists have begun to express concern over the effects of environmental pollution and chemical exposure on human health, specifically, reproductive health.

Our homes, our relationships, our workplaces, and our lifestyles are small units functioning within a greater, more global environment. The "purity" of each unit determines its ability to safeguard our mental, spiritual, and physical health. A pure unit is one in which we can thrive. If one or more of these units that make up our living environment becomes impure for whatever reason, our ability to thrive is compromised.

Unfortunately, modern lifestyles often cause us to compromise on a daily basis. For instance, we compromise our physical well-being each time we take a breath of polluted air or consume food that has been tainted with pesticides or preservatives. We may compromise our emotional and physical well-being through stressors we encounter at work or at home. Even maneuvering through traffic or waiting on lines at the bank can be stressful. While some harmful factors of modern life are unavoidable, we do have choices.

Purifying the units of our environment can be difficult and time-consuming. To completely eliminate all of the detriments that surround us would require such a strict and drastic change in our lifestyle that most of us would be unwilling or unable to do so. We can, however, strive toward a purer way of life by changing those aspects of our lives over which we do have control.

ENVIRONMENTAL FACTORS

Recent research in the area of environmental pollution and human health has highlighted growing concern over the proliferation of chemicals that are ending up in our food, water, air, and soil. Of particular concern are the effects of endocrine-disrupting chemicals, also known as *xenobiotics*, on human reproduction.

Capable of imitating the hormone estrogen in both males and females, xenobiotics attach themselves to estrogen receptors in the body. Normally, the body's own estrogen attaches to these receptors. When these foreign "estrogen mimickers" enter the body (either through food, water, air, or skin contact), they begin to "crowd out" natural estrogen. Xenobiotics are believed to be capable of disrupting female menstrual cycles, altering hormone levels, causing miscarriages, and damaging ova and sperm.

There are currently sixty-seven known endocrine-disrupting chemicals, including dioxins, PCBs (polychlorinated biphenyls), and DDT (dicholordiphenyltrichloroethane). They are present in products as diverse as pesticides, fertilizers, plastics, waste incineration, and electrical equipment. (Keep in mind that although we know of sixty-seven, there may be hundreds or even thousands more.) And although many of these toxins have been banned for use in this country—some for many years—they are still around.

Once endocrine-disrupting chemicals find their way into the environment, through, for example, direct waste disposal or as a byproduct of some industrial process, they tend to remain for a very long time. Unlike organic substances that break down in the environment, these toxins *bio-accumulate*— move their way up the food chain. Eventually, many are consumed by animals and humans.

Although our knowledge of the effects of endocrine-disrupters on human reproduction is still developing, animal studies have shown them to be damaging. Animals throughout the world, and particularly in areas where pollution levels are the highest, have been suffering severe reproductive consequences for decades. For instance, high levels of PCBs off the coast of Mexico are believed to be responsible for the reproductive failures of marine animals such as dolphins. Because dolphins and humans are genetically similar, scientists believe that PCB pollution may be as detrimental to human reproductive health as it is to that of the dolphins.

In Norway, exposure to toxic chemicals such as PCBs and DDT have been implicated in the increased number of congenital reproductive system defects in polar bears. The list of toxin-exposed animals born with such defects is long. This is probably our greatest warning that all is not well.

Unfortunately, our knowledge of the reproductive toxicity of many chemicals is either unknown or incomplete. In 1996, the United States Environmental Protection Agency (EPA) began to expand its research on these endocrine disrupters to determine their effects on human reproduction. It took on the daunting task of screening approximately 62,000 chemicals for endocrine-disrupting capabilities. The aim of the project is to determine which chemicals in our environment are responsible for endometriosis, cancer, hormone imbalances, and fibroids in women, and prostate cancer, lowered testosterone levels, and decreasing sperm counts in men. (In 1992, a team of Danish reproductive specialists announced that since 1938, male sperm counts in the industrialized world have dropped by approximately 50 percent.)

A recent study completed by the Department of Preventive Medicine and Environmental Health at the University of Iowa College of Medicine, involved the reproductive health of women. The study examined the impact of pesticides, including DDT, on human reproductive systems. (Although DDT has been banned in the United States since 1972, it still lingers in the environment.) The study found that women who are regularly exposed to pesticides are up to three times more likely to become infertile than women who are not in contact with these environmental hazards. The effects of these endocrine disrupters on men are only now being studied.

OCCUPATIONAL EXPOSURE TO HARMFUL ELEMENTS

A 1994 article that appeared in the *Journal of the American Industrial Hygiene Association* stated that disorders of reproduction and infertility are among the top ten work-related conditions in the United States. Men and women who work in industries that manufacture or use certain chemicals such as benzene and xylene, or elements such as mercury and lead, should be aware of their link to impaired reproductive function. Anyone exposed to these substances in his or her living environment is also at risk. Because exposure generally occurs on a daily basis, the side effects are cumulative and often long term. For this reason, awareness is critical.

Table 3.1 includes a list of some of these hazardous materials, their effects on reproduction, and those who are most at risk. Anyone exposed to these elements should be aware of

Table 3.1. Occupational Hazards and Reproductive Health

Material	Common Sources	Possible Effects on Reproduction	Those at High Risk
Benzene	Rubber, lubricants, dyes, detergents, and pesticides	• sperm abnormalities, including low sperm count • irregular menstrual cycles • abnormal ovulatory function	• workers who produce or use solvents, plastics, rubber, glues, dyes, or detergents • agricultural workers
Estrogen, synthetic	Birth control pills, fertility medication	• hormone imbalance • increased infertility in women	• pharmaceutical workers involved in the manufacture of synthetic hormones • farmers who administer hormones to livestock
Lead	Leaded paints, ceramic glues, batteries, hair colorants	• increased infertility in both men and women • increased risk of miscarriage • low sperm counts	• auto workers • ceramic and pottery makers • electronics workers • farmers
Mercury	Batteries, dental amalgams, agricultural fungicides, thermometers	• decreased reproductive function due to accumulation in ovarian tissue	• dental workers • battery makers • commercial fishermen • employees working with pesticides
Nitrous oxide ("laughing gas")	Common anesthetic	• sperm abnormalities • increased risk of miscarriage	• health care workers in dental clinics and hospitals • veterinary surgeons • animal lab researchers
Xylene	Paints, paint thinners, and varnishes	• decreased ovarian size • irregular menstrual cycles	• auto garage workers • painters • wood-processing plant workers • furniture refinishers

the risks and make sure that the highest safety standards are maintained to minimize these dangers. In general, those who are trying to conceive should reduce their exposure as much as possible.

The Agency for Toxic Substances and Disease Registry in Atlanta, Georgia, is a good source for further information on hazardous substances and their related illnesses. You can contact the agency at 1–888–422–8737.

Let's take a closer look at some of these environmental hazards and their possible links to impaired reproduction.

Lead

Lead is a particularly worrisome toxic metallic element because of its abundance in our environment. Once lead enters the human body, it travels to the brain, central nervous system, and glands, where it accumulates. Among other health problems, lead exposure has been linked to decreased fertility, higher rates of miscarriage, and low sperm counts. Major sources of lead include lead-based paint (usually found in homes built before 1980), ceramic items coated with leaded glaze (common in ceramicware from China, Mexico, and Italy), leaded gasoline, batteries, hair colorant, tap water, and waste incineration. If you are exposed to any of these lead sources on a regular basis, you should be checked periodically for lead accumulation. This can be done through a simple hair analysis or blood test.

Eating high-fiber foods, such as apples and bran, can help flush common environmental toxins, including lead and other heavy metals, from your system. Chelation therapy (see the inset on page 39) is another effective procedure for toxic elimination.

Xylene

Xylene is a colorless, sweet-smelling petroleum product commonly used as a solvent in the printing, rubber, and leather industries. Also found in paint thinners and varnishes, xylene is one of the top thirty chemicals produced in the United States in terms of volume. While xylene does break down in the environment quickly (unlike dioxins and other chemicals), daily exposure to high levels (more than 100 parts per million of xylene) may cause infertility in women.

Chelation Therapy

Chelation therapy has been growing in popularity since the 1940s, when it was first discovered that ethylenediamintetracetic acid (EDTA), a synthetic amino acid, could be used as a treatment for a number of medical conditions, including arteriosclerosis (hardening of the arteries) and heavy metal poisoning. EDTA acts like an antioxidant, ridding the body of dangerous heavy metals, restoring enzyme function, and controlling free radical activity.

EDTA is administered to patients intravenously under the supervision of a physician. It works by chelating (binding to) saturated fats and toxic metals such as lead or mercury, then flushing them out of the body through the kidneys. Each chelation treatment consists of 3 to 4 grams of EDTA, and takes about four hours to administer.

Used in conjunction with lifestyle and dietary changes that reduce exposure to toxic chemicals and increase nutrient-rich food, chelation therapy is considered a safe way to detoxify the body. The procedure, which has not had one fatality in over fifty years of administration, has been approved by the American Medical Association for the purpose of heavy metal detoxification.

Benzene

Derived from petroleum, benzene is a colorless, sweet-smelling liquid. It is widely manufactured in the United States and used by industries in the manufacturing of rubber, lubricants, dyes, detergents, and pesticides. The air surrounding gas stations and hazardous waste sites contains moderately high levels of benzene. (The EPA has found high levels of benzene in at least 813 of the 1,430 hazardous waste sites throughout the United States.)

A 1998 study, conducted by the National Institute of Occupational Health in Norway, found a connection between benzopyrene (car exhaust) and ovulation failure in laboratory animals.

Women who are continually exposed to high levels of benzene may develop irregular menstrual cycles and experience a decrease in the size of their ovaries, causing an increased risk of infertility. Women who work in an environment where benzene is used to manufacture products such as plastics, nylon, synthetic fibers, pesticides, and resins are at greatest risk. A simple blood test can check for the presence of this chemical.

Nitrous oxide

Nitrous oxide, also known as "laughing gas," is a commonly used anesthetic in dentistry and surgery. Numerous studies have found that dental workers who are constantly exposed to nitrous oxide have more than twice as many infertility problems as the general population. These problems include increased incidents of miscarriage and sperm abnormalities.

Mercury

Mercury is a highly poisonous heavy metal that is implicated in a wide range of health problems, including neurological damage. Regular exposure to mercury, an estrogen-mimicking metal, may also cause impaired ovarian function in women.

Dental workers, battery makers, and commercial fishermen are often exposed to mercury, which is used in dental amalgams, agricultural fungicides, antiseptics, and thermometers. According to the environmental protection agency, the average American may not even be aware that he or she is at risk for mercury poisoning. In the agency's 1997 report entitled *The Mercury Report to Congress,* the greatest sources of mercury pollution in our environment come from coal-fired power plants, waste incinerators, and medical waste. Anyone living near these sources has reason to be concerned.

In addition, freshwater fish, particularly those from the Great Lakes and smaller lakes located in the Midwest, may be equally dangerous. Northern pike, trout, and walleye are particularly suspect.

Pesticides

Due to their widespread use, pesticides have been a health concern for decades. Each year sees an estimated 45,000 cases worldwide of pesticide poisoning. In addition, pesticides have been implicated in an increased number of impaired reproductive functions and fetal damage in both animals and humans.

Pesticides are present in the ground, in the air, and in our food and water supplies. Especially in the Midwestern United States, high concentrations of pesticides have leached into the groundwater—one EPA report in the 1980s revealed seventeen different types of pesticides and herbicides in the groundwater of twenty-three states. While the EPA has been given the onerous task of tracking the presence of hazardous wastes in our environment, and a government fund has been established to clean up the chemicals, in fact, no one knows the enormity of the problem. Many areas of the country still

Beware Those Fruits and Vegetables

Many of the pesticides that are banned in the United States are still used on fruits and vegetables grown outside the country. Ironically, we import much of this pesticide-laden produce, which winds up on our supermarket shelves. To help protect yourself against pesticides that are commonly found on or in foods:

- *Whenever possible, purchase organically grown produce.*

- *Do not eat imported produce, which may have been treated with pesticides that have been banned in the United States.*

- *Discard the outer leaves of leafy vegetables such as cabbage and lettuce. They can contain the bulk of the pesticide residue.*

- *Peel produce or scrub it with liquid detergent and warm water. Scrubbing can remove about 40 percent of surface pesticide residue.*

contain hazardous wastes that include these harmful chemicals.

The effects of pesticides on reproductive health have not been studied sufficiently on human beings to determine the true extent of their damage. However, it is known that pesticides such as carbaryl (sevin) and 2,4-D, still used widely throughout the world, can damage and reduce sperm levels. And solvents such as benzene and xylene, found in a number of pesticide formulations, have been implicated in reproductive disorders in women. The University of Iowa College of Medicine study, discussed earlier, concluded that women who are exposed to pesticides regularly may face a 3.02 times greater risk of developing ovulatory problems. Of particular concern is the presence of "endocrine disrupting" organo-chlorines.

Organochlorines

Organochlorines are a family of organic chemicals that have chlorine atoms within their molecular structure. They have been used throughout the world as insecticides such as DDT, and industrial chemicals like PCBs. Some organochlorines, such as dioxins, are byproducts of industrial processes. Being biologically stable, organichlorines do not break down once they are released into the environment. Instead, they bio-accumulate and eventually work their way up the food chain. Organochlorine deposits have been found in human and animal fat. They are extremely toxic and potentially carcinogenic.

There is increasing concern over the amount of organochlorines that are present in our environment, and their long-term effects on human reproduction, as well as on overall health. Much of this concern is because organochlorines are estrogen mimickers. Scientists now widely suspect that by attaching to estrogen receptors in the human body, organochlorines can disrupt the natural hormonal balance of both male and female reproductive systems. As such, organochlorines have been implicated in conditions such as endometriosis, ovarian failure, and lowered sperm counts.

One study that appeared in the October 1995 issue of *Environmental Health Perspectives* details the effects of dioxins on female rhesus monkeys. The monkeys, who had been exposed to dioxins for four years, developed endometriosis. According to a 1993 Greenpeace report, *Chlorine, Human Health and the Environment: The Breast Cancer Warning*, organochlorines can "cause reproductive and developmental impairment, hormonal disruptions, genetic mutations, cancer, birth defects . . . and damage to the liver." The liver maintains a proper balance between male and female hormones in the body. Liver damage can cause increased estrogen levels, resulting in infertility.

A growing number of scientists and environmentalists are warning of a potential human reproduction apocalypse if the amount of organochlorines to which we are exposed, continues to increase. The main infertility concern lies in the capability of organochlorines to disrupt the female hormone estrogen, causing harm to the reproductive system. Let's take a closer look at DDT and PCBs, and their effects on fertility.

DDT

Dicholordiphenyltrichloroethane (DDT), an endocrine disrupter, was used heavily as an agricultural pesticide in the United States until it was banned in the 1970s. However, because it bio-accumulates, DDT is still present in the environment. A Natural Resources Defense Council survey found that these pesticides are still turning up in our fruits, vegetables, and water supply.

DDT has been shown to impair the reproductive systems of marine life in areas where it was once heavily used. At the 1994 Symposium on Estrogens in the Environment, one research paper stated that, "there are reports of wildlife being exposed to the pesticide DDT, which produced male infertility resulting from low sperm counts."

If DDT's effects on human reproduction are even remotely similar, we, as human beings, have much reason to be concerned.

PCBs

Polychlorinated biphenyls (PCBs) are a family of more than 200 chemical compounds. Between 1929 (when they were first manufactured) and 1979 (when they were finally banned in the United States due to their link with cancer), an estimated 1.1 billion pounds of PCBs were produced as coolants, lubricants, and insulating fluids. Until that point, however, they had been freely disposed of in lakes and open landfills that were close to rivers and harbors throughout North America.

Unfortunately, PCBs, like DDT, were able to leak into inland and coastal waters, polluting the water supplies of surrounding communities. While the exact effects on human reproduction are not known, PCBs are suspected of being endocrine disruptors, with the ability to throw hormone levels (including reproductive hormones) off balance.

Consumers Union reported in 1992 that in a study of fish in retail markets in Chicago and New York, PCBs were present in nearly 43 percent of the salmon, 50 percent of the whitefish, and 25 percent of the swordfish. (This same study discovered that DDT continued to show up in 334 of 386 domestic fish samples over ten years after the chemical had been banned.) A growing number of scientists and environmentalists are warning of a potential human reproduction apocalypse if the amount of organochlorines that we are exposed to continues to increase.

Although your ability to control exposure to organochlorines is limited, you can take the following steps to minimize the possible risks:

❑ Avoid drinking chlorinated tap water. Instead drink bottled water that has been filtered of chemicals and chlorine.

❑ Choose organic fruits and vegetables, which have been cultivated without chemical fertilizers and pesticides.

❑ When eating meat, fish, or poultry, be sure to remove all fat. Pesticides and other toxins accumulate in fatty tissue. If possible, choose beef and chicken from organically raised animals.

❑ Eat minimal amounts of coastal or freshwater fish, including salmon, herring, swordfish, bluefish, yellow or white perch, trout, whitefish, catfish, or carp. Select fish that live in deep waters. The safest offshore fish to eat are cod, scrod, flounder, haddock, pollock, sole, and yellowfin tuna. The next safest fish include hake, halibut, ocean perch, pompano, albacore tuna, and tilefish.

❏ Whenever possible, choose younger (smaller) fish; they are more likely to have accumulated fewer toxins in their shorter lifetimes.

❏ After cooking fish, trim away any dark meat and the tail, which are the fattiest tissues.

Our understanding of the effects of chemical toxicity on human reproduction is gradually increasing as greater efforts are now being made in the Western world to research this field. However, the responsibility ultimately lies with each individual to become further aware and further involved; to know the risks; and to take the necessary steps to protect themselves from potentially harmful chemicals.

LIFESTYLE FACTORS

Women in the Western world have come a long way since the 1950s. In business, government, sports, and education—areas once dominated by men—women have risen to important and influential levels. More women than ever before are working outside the home, and salary and education level disparities between men and women are slowly shrinking. The opportunities now available to women are seemingly endless and full of hope. However, advancement and equal opportunity haven't come without a downside—stress and anxiety.

Many women struggle to be everything to everyone—wives, mothers, employees, employers. Often they find themselves with precious little time to care for their own needs. They are often caught up in a number of harmful features common to today's modern lifestyle, including increased stress levels, lack of exercise, overuse of medication, consumption of caffeine and alcohol, and the use of cigarettes. Over time, these wreak havoc on immune systems, reproductive systems, and general good health.

Alcohol Consumption

Women who are trying to become pregnant should avoid alcoholic beverages both prior to and after conception. During pregnancy, alcohol consumption increases a woman's risk of giving birth to a child with fetal alcohol syndrome (FAS). Typically, FAS babies have a number of physical and mental deficiencies. At birth, they are generally underweight and smaller than normal infants. Characteristically, their faces are somewhat malformed with low nasal bridges and thin upper lips, and many have heart and joint abnormalities. Mental retardation, poor coordination, and behavioral problems are the most serious mental defects affecting children with FAS. Even though much research on FAS has been done, it is still not known how much alcohol during pregnancy is safe, and if certain alcoholic drinks are "safer" than others. For this reason, women who are pregnant should refrain from drinking any amount of alcohol (especially during the first trimester).

In addition to causing possible damage to the fetus, alcohol consumption can also impair fertility. A number of studies have indicated that consuming large amounts of alcohol can prevent ovulation, as well as increase the incidence of miscarriage. One study conducted by Harvard University researchers found that women who consumed in excess of seven drinks a week were more likely to be infertile due to ovulation problems than women who did not drink. The study also indicated that women who consume between four and seven drinks a week have a 30 percent increased risk of infertility. And men who drink on a regular basis were found to have a higher than average percentage of abnormal sperm.

Alcohol has also been implicated in causing elevated pro-

lactin levels. As seen in Chapter 1, prolactin is a hormone produced by the anterior pituitary gland (the same gland that produces luteinizing and follicle-stimulating hormones). In males,
high levels of prolactin can lower testosterone levels, reducing
sperm production. In women, high prolactin levels, or *hyper-
prolactinaemia,* can cause irregular ovulation and menstrual
cycles, and lower progesterone levels. Without adequate progesterone, the uterine wall cannot maintain an endometrial lining that is adequate enough to house a fertilized egg.

Given the well-documented and conclusive evidence link-
ing alcohol consumption with infertility, if you drink regularly and are having trouble conceiving, there may be a link
between the two.

Cigarette Smoking

A Toronto research team found that cotinine, a chemical present in cigarette smoke, collects in the ovaries of women who
are exposed to it. The researchers concluded that this chemical
may affect the development and viability of ova. Naturally,
the more a woman smokes, the more cotinine collects in her
ovaries. Even nonsmokers can be affected if they are constantly exposed to second-hand smoke.

A study performed in 1985 by the National Institute of
Environmental Health in North Carolina, found that female
smokers were 3 to 4 times more likely than non-smokers to
experience delays in conception. While other factors, such as
stress, poor diet, and alcohol consumption, should not be
ignored for the part they play in increasing infertility odds,
cigarette smoking can be a real culprit.

According to one study that was conducted at the
University of North Carolina in 1994, men who smoke produce an average of 13 to 17 percent less sperm than non-
smokers. And in another study that appeared in a 1981 issue
of *Lancet,* male smokers tend also to have more abnormal
sperm than nonsmokers.

Caffeine

Caffeine has been found to have a possible negative effect on the fertility of both men and women. Numerous studies have indicated that men who drink moderate to large amounts of caffeinated coffee daily (three or more cups) have lower sperm counts and weaker sperm motility than men who drink little or no coffee.

A 1992 study conducted by the Yale University School of Medicine involved 1,909 women and studied the effects of caffeine consumption on fertility. The study found that the more coffee the women consumed, the more difficult it was for them to conceive. Compared to a group of women who did not drink caffeinated coffee, the women who regularly drank one cup per day showed a 55 percent higher chance of conception difficulty. Those women who drank more than three cups a day had a 176 percent higher chance of conception failure. Caffeine consumption during pregnancy is also discouraged, as it may be linked to increased risk of miscarriage.

The reason caffeine appears to have an impact on conception and pregnancy is not certain. One theory, however, suggests that caffeine can alter hormone levels. Such an imbalance can affect ovulation in women, and sperm production in men.

Overexercising

While proper exercise is important for a healthy cardiovascular system and toned muscles, too much exercise can actually reduce hormone levels and cause ovulation to cease. A number of female athletes involved with endurance sports, such as long-distance running and gymnastics, have reported that their menstrual periods were infrequent or stopped altogether at the onset of rigorous athletic training.

Women who exercise heavily and are finding it difficult to conceive should reduce their physical activity substantially. This will help them regain a normal menstrual cycle.

Improper Weight Levels

It is important to stay within your proper weight range when trying to conceive. A drop of 10 to 15 percent below your ideal body weight can interfere with fertility. A woman should have at least 22 percent body fat to maintain ovulation. As such, women who are underweight or who have an eating disorder such as anorexia nervosa or bulimia may stop ovulating.

Conversely, women who are severely overweight and do not exercise often have very high estrogen levels. This increases their risk of becoming anovulatory. Extremely high or low body weight is believed to be the cause in as much as 12 percent of infertility cases.

There are a number of ways to determine your healthiest weight, and to discover if, by current standards, you are overweight or underweight. One of the simplest means used by professionals is the body mass index (BMI), which describes body weight in relation to height. Simply put, as a person's weight increases, so does his or her BMI.

You can easily determine your own BMI by using the following formula:

$$\frac{\text{Weight (pounds)}}{\text{Height (inches)}^2} \times 705 = \text{BMI}$$

To use this formula, just follow these steps. Let's assume, for the sake of this example, that you are 5 feet 4 inches tall and weigh 121 pounds.

1. First, calculate your height in inches, and square it—in other words, multiply the number by itself. In our example, your height (5 feet 4 inches) is 64 inches. So:

$$64 \times 64 = 4,096$$

2. Now, determine your weight in pounds. In our example, your weight is 121 pounds.

3. Divide the smaller number (in this case, 121) by the larger number (4,096), rounding off your answer to the nearest hundredth:

$$121 \div 4,096 = .03$$

4. Multiply your final number by 705.

$$.03 \times 705 = 21$$

In this example, your BMI is 21. Don't have a calculator on hand? The following chart will help you determine your BMI at a glance.

Body Mass Index

BMI	20	21	22	23	24	25	26	27	28	29	30
Height					Weight in Pounds						
5'0"	102	107	112	117	122	127	132	138	143	148	153
5'1"	106	111	117	122	127	132	138	143	148	154	159
5'2"	109	114	120	125	130	135	141	146	152	158	163
5'3"	113	119	124	130	135	141	146	152	158	164	169
5'4"	117	123	129	135	141	146	152	158	164	170	176
5'5"	120	126	132	138	144	150	156	162	168	174	180
5'6"	124	131	137	143	149	156	162	168	174	180	187
5'7"	127	134	140	147	153	159	166	172	178	185	191
5'8"	132	139	145	152	158	165	172	178	185	191	198
5'9"	135	142	149	155	162	169	176	182	189	196	203
5'10"	140	147	154	161	168	175	182	189	196	203	210
5'11"	143	150	157	164	171	179	186	193	200	207	214
6'0"	148	155	162	170	177	185	192	199	207	214	221
6'1"	151	158	166	174	181	189	196	204	211	219	226
6'2"	156	164	171	179	187	195	203	210	218	226	234
6'3"	159	167	175	183	191	199	207	215	223	231	239
6'4"	164	172	181	189	197	205	214	222	230	238	246

Source: Centers for Disease Control; Department of Agriculture.

In general, BMIs between 19 and 24.9 are considered optimal. A BMI of 25 to 29.9 is considered overweight, while an index of 30 or more is considered obese.

If you are very muscular and/or have dense bones, your BMI is likely to be higher than the standards recommend. This does not necessarily mean that you are overweight. If you fall into this category, you can get a better idea of what your ideal body weight should be by having your percentage of body fat measured. A health professional such as an exercise physiologist or nutritionist can do this for you.

Stress

Stress may contribute to infertility by altering hormone levels in the body, particularly progesterone. As you know, progesterone is important in maintaining the uterine lining. Without a proper lining, a fertilized egg cannot remain implanted.

In 1996, Sam Wasser of the University of Washington in Seattle conducted a study on yellow baboons in Tanzania. He found that stress in their environment plays a major role in the fertility of these baboons, whose physiology closely resembles that of humans. Wasser found that during stressful dry seasons, progesterone levels in the female baboons dropped, preventing them from sustaining a pregnancy. During the rainy season, however, their progesterone levels normalized and fertility rates rose. Wasser argues that if stressors in the environment of the yellow baboon can influence hormone balance and fertility patterns, then stressors in our environment may affect human infertility as well.

Most of us live in a stress-filled world. We feel pressure and anxiety over financial concerns and work responsibilities, as well as frustrations when we find ourselves caught in traffic jams or long lines at the bank or grocery store. Such everyday stressors are countless, indeed, and may seem impossible to eliminate. We must, however, strive to slow down this hectic pace.

When preparing the body for conception and pregnancy, it is best to be calm and relaxed both physically and mentally. Possible ways in which a sense of relaxation and tranquility can be achieved include reducing work hours, taking regular vacations, setting aside some time each day to be alone with your thoughts, spending time alone with your partner, and incorporating stress-reducing practices such as meditation or massage into your routine. Many people find that some form of meditation allows them to relax and unwind, enabling them to cope better with life's daily challenges. The antistress relaxation techniques presented in Chapter 8 are particularly helpful for those who lead stress-filled lives and are having problems conceiving.

Medications

A few medications, if taken regularly and for long periods of time, can have a negative effect on the reproductive systems of both women and men. If you are having difficulty conceiving and have been taking any of the medications listed below, chances are there may be a connection.

Medications are prescribed for a reason. Do not stop taking a medicine arbitrarily without first consulting your physician. He or she may be able to prescribe an alternative, preferably natural, treatment. In many cases, alternative medicine can be used in conjunction with traditional medication. In other words, a specific herb or combination of herbs may be able to counterbalance the negative effects of the medication you are taking. In this instance, consulting the services of a naturopath can be very helpful.

Antihistamines

Used to help relieve the symptoms of allergies and head colds, antihistamines are sold over-the-counter and taken by millions of people each year. When taken for an extended period of time, antihistamines can change the texture and quantity of cervical mucus, making it more difficult for sperm to make their way to the uterus.

Non-Steroidal Anti-Inflammatory Drugs

Non-steroidal anti-inflammatory drugs (NSAIDs), such as ibuprofen (Advil, Motrin, and Nuprin), and naproxen (Anaprox, Naprosyn, and Aleve) are often used to reduce specific inflammations of the joints and muscles, the pain of arthritis, and the discomfort of menstrual cramps. Overuse of these drugs, however, can also inhibit ovulation during the menstrual cycle, making conception difficult if not impossible.

Two 1996 studies, published in the *British Journal of Rheumatology,* indicate a link between the regular use of NSAIDs with an increased incidence of *unruptured follicle syndrome.* This condition is caused by a lack of luteinizing hormone, which prevents follicles in the ovaries from releasing their eggs.

High Blood Pressure Medication

Drugs used to treat high blood pressure (hypertension), such as reserpine and alpha methyldopa, can increase prolactin production in women. A hormone released by the pituitary gland during pregnancy, prolactin stimulates the breasts to produce milk. Elevated prolactin levels often cause ovulation to stop. Symptoms include a lack of or infrequent menstrual periods, sore and painful breasts, and the production of breast milk in non-nursing women.

Exposure to Electromagnetic Fields

Most people never give a second thought to the safety of their electric clock radios, sewing machines, or televisions. But such electrical sources emit invisible non-ionizing radiation that is generated by electromagnetic fields (EMFs). Constant low-level exposure to EMFs has been implicated in endometriosis and miscarriages, as well as a number of other serious health conditions, including chronic fatigue syndrome, memory loss, and certain cancers. To understand what an electromagnetic field is, first it is important to understand the difference between a natural and an artificial field.

Natural fields that generate both electric and magnetic radiation are generated by the planets, the sun, the moon, and by every living thing, including our own bodies. Our bodies are regulated and attuned to the Earth's field, and they pulse at about the same rate. However, artificial electromagnetic fields pulse at a different rate. These waves radiate from just about everything connected to an electrical circuit, including computers and computer monitors, telephone lines, microwave ovens, electric blankets, electric clocks, televisions, and hair dryers. The currents in these pulsating waves move back and forth in an alternating pattern. And it is this movement that may be interfering with the body's own electrical current, disturbing cell membranes.

Both the strength of the electromagnetic field and the duration of exposure are believed to influence health, including reproductive health. According to a study conducted by the University of Iowa College of Medicine, women who regularly find themselves in close proximity to computer monitors are up to three times more likely to experience endometriosis and cervical abnormalities than women who are not. In addition, long-time exposure to EMFs has been implicated in higher incidences of miscarriage. They also may be linked to certain cancers and may exacerbate pre-existing conditions such as Parkinson's disease and certain mental disorders such as depression.

To reduce your odds against exposure to electromagnetic fields, especially if you are trying to get pregnant, consider the following suggestions:

❑ Distance yourself from EMF sources. Keep a distance of at least six feet or more from television sets, refrigerators, freezers, and electrical heaters, and at least one foot from hair dryers. Sit two to three feet from the front of computer monitors.

❏ Use an EMF shield for computer monitors as well as television sets. Sold in electronics stores, these shields can help reduce harmful emissions.

❏ Do not use electric blankets.

❏ Whenever possible, use battery-operated appliances rather than electric ones.

Remember, while it is impossible to completely avoid non-ionizing rays generated by electromagnetic fields, you can do something about lowering your exposure to them. Prudent avoidance is the key.

SUMMING IT UP

Counterbalancing the damage done to our bodies by chemicals and environmental toxins, alcohol consumption, cigarette smoke, and stress clearly is not easy. Depending on where you live and work and the type of lifestyle you lead, you are likely exposed to a wide number of potentially toxic environmental and lifestyle factors each day. Eliminating or at least reducing your exposure to these factors is helpful to your reproductive health and good health in general.

In order to strengthen the reproductive system and encourage fertility, try to "purify" your immediate living environment as much as possible. Try to reduce or eliminate factors that may be affecting your fertility—stress, chemical exposure and exposure to electromagnetic fields, alcohol consumption, and cigarette smoke. Not only will such measures increase your likelihood of conceiving, they will also help improve your overall mental and physical health. You should also eat a healthy diet. As you will see in the next chapters, eating nutritional enzyme-rich foods, such as asparagus, celery, and dandelions, especially in their fresh raw state, helps detoxify and cleanse the system.

4

Foods and Fertility

While it's no secret that proper dietary nutrition is important for maintaining good health, it's not as well known that certain foods and nutrients can negatively influence conception and reproductive health. The damaging effects of xenobiotics—endocrine-disrupting chemicals—on reproduction were discussed in the previous chapter. This chapter presents the effects of *phytoestrogens*—plant-based estrogens—as well as xenobiotic hormones, and some nonestrogenic foods on reproductive system function. If you find that some of these foods are typically found in your diet, don't panic! The aim of this information is not to create a sense of fear, but rather to increase your awareness and recommend that you practice prudence in your consumption of these foods.

PHYTOESTROGENS

Phytoestrogens are weak estrogenic compounds that occur naturally in a number of edible plants, including fruits, vegetables, and herbs. Two well known phytoestrogens include *genistein*, found in soy beans, and *cuomestrol*, a very potent phytoestrogen found in alfalfa. Numerous animal studies and our knowledge of the role of estrogen on the reproductive system indicate that high levels of phytoestrogens (such as the xenobiotic endocrine-disrupting chemicals discussed in Chapter 3) are capable of mimicking natural estrogen and attaching themselves to estrogen receptors throughout the body. Because the menstrual cycle relies on the timely and balanced release of hormones—as estrogen production increases, follicle stimulating hormone (FSH) production decreases. When excessive amounts of phytoestrogens are present during the first half of the menstrual cycle, estrogen levels in the blood soar. This "turns off" the production of FSH, which, in turn, prevents an egg from maturing. In fact, continuously high levels of phytoestrogens are capable of preventing ovulation and implantation of an embryo. Some scientists have considered that phytoestrogens act as a natural form of birth control.

Many studies have been conducted on the consumption of phytoestrogenic foods and their effects on the reproductive function of animals. In a few instances, the side effects have been very dramatic. One study observed that livestock who were fed steady diets of alfalfa, which contains the potent phytoestrogen, coumestrol, had increased incidents of misshapen uteri. In another study conducted in 1997 by the Departments of Animal Science, Food and Nutrition at Southern Illinois University, female laboratory rats were fed a diet high in soy protein, which contains high levels of the phytoestrogen genistein. As a result, the rats showed a decrease in the number of ovarian follicles.

It is important to take into consideration that, with few exceptions, studies that investigate the link between phytoestrogens and fertility have involved animals, mainly laboratory rats and livestock, not humans. Also, the amount of phytoestrogens typically consumed by livestock is many times greater than the amount of phytoestrogens consumed by humans. The diet of pigs, for instance, typically consists of 20 percent phytoestrogenic soy meal—much higher than the average soy consumption found in a typical Western diet. On the other hand, preliminary studies in 1996 involving women who were given a diet high in phytoestrogen-containing foods, did indicate that this diet significantly lengthened the menstrual cycle, making it more difficult to determine time of ovulation.

Let's take a closer look at some of these phytoestrogenic foods and their possible impact on reproduction.

Soy Products

Soy products, including soy milk, tempeh, and tofu, have long been staples in the Far Eastern diet. Since the 1970s, the popularity of these foods has increased in the United States, particularly among vegetarians. The reason? Soy beans are high in protein, iron, and calcium, and low in saturated fat and sodium. However, soy is also rich in the phytoestrogen genistein.

As mentioned earlier, studies on laboratory rats have indicated that high soy diets can affect reproductive function by decreasing the number of ovarian follicles. Another study conducted in 1994 by the Dunn Clinical Nutrition Center in Cambridge, England, found that women who consumed 60 grams of tofu daily for one month experienced an increase in the length of their menstrual cycles. Such changes make it more difficult to determine when ovulation will occur.

More research on the effects of soy products needs to be done before a more definitive conclusion regarding their effects on the reproductive system can be made. However, it may be wise to recommend that women who eat lots of soy products and have erratic menstrual cycles limit their intake of these foods.

Peas

In 1949, Indian scientist Dr. S.N. Sanyal began a study on the contraceptive effect of green peas *(Pisum sativum)*. This study was based on his theory that overconsumption of this legume, a staple of the Tibetan diet, had caused that country's population growth to stay stable for 200 years.

Dr. Sanyal was able to isolate the peas' estrogenic chemical compound *m-xylohydroquinone* and concentrate it into a capsule. When the women in the study consumed the capsules daily over a period of a few months, fertility decreased 50 to 60 percent. Men who followed the same regimen experienced a noticeable drop in sperm counts. Dr. Sanyal concluded that m-xylohydroquinone had the ability to control progesterone and estrogen production in the human body. Based on the anti-fertility effects of green peas, consumption of this legume should be avoided by couples who are trying to become pregnant.

High levels of phytoestrogens are found in a number of foods, including:

Alfalfa	Basil	Garlic	Potatoes
Anise	Carrots	Ginseng	Rice
Apples	Cherries	Green beans	Sesame
Barley	Fennel	Peas	Soy

As the effects of phytoestrogen-containing foods is still not clear, it may be best not to build a diet solely around them. Couples who are trying to conceive might consider eating these foods in moderation—no more than one serving daily. Women who already have high estrogen levels and experience anovulatory problems may be wise to avoid these foods altogether. And, as seen in Chapter 5, they should supplement their diets with omega-3 fatty acids and estrogen-balancing herbs.

XENOBIOTIC HORMONES

Xenobiotic hormones—estrogenic substances derived from plants—have long been added to the feed of cattle, poultry, and pigs. These hormones are typically injected into these animals to increase their weight and encourage tenderness. In turn, we consume these hormones whenever we eat the meat from an animal that has been injected with them.

In itself, eating meat or eggs that contain trace amounts of estrogen does not cause infertility; however, the effects of estrogen exposure are cumulative. A steady diet of eggs and meat will increase the amount of estrogen absorbed by the body. This quickly binds to estrogen receptors, raising blood estrogen levels. A high-fat diet and the consumption of alcohol compounds the problem even further, as fats and alcohol put an extra strain on the liver, making it more difficult to flush the extra estrogen from the body.

Clearly, the best way to avoid xenobiotic hormones is simply not to eat them. Whenever possible, choose meat from organically raised cattle and chickens—they are free of estrogenic hormones. Eggs from organically raised chickens are available in most supermarkets. Meat from organically raised animals is a bit more difficult to find, but it is sold in a small number of health food stores.

NON-ESTROGENIC FOODS

In addition to the estrogen-containing food products listed earlier, there are a number of other foods that are well known for their "anti-fertility" effects. These foods do not contain estrogen mimickers; however, they do contain chemical compounds that are toxic to sperm and ova. *Galactose*, a sugar found in milk, is toxic to ova, while *Gossypium hirsutum*, present in cottonseed oil, and the alkaloid caffeine, are known to affect sperm production in men. Therefore, milk products, cottonseed oil, and beverages containing caffeine should be avoided by those who are trying to conceive.

Coffee and Other Caffeinated Beverages

As seen in Chapter 3, coffee and other caffeinated beverages can affect fertility in both men and women. Numerous studies on caffeine have indicated that men who drink moderate to large amounts of coffee (three or more cups a day) have lower sperm counts and weaker sperm motility than men who drink little or no coffee. Other studies have shown an increased chance of conception failure among women who drink more than three cups of coffee daily. And high coffee consumption among pregnant women has been linked to an increased risk of miscarriage.

Milk

Women who suffer from unexplained infertility may want to look at their consumption of dairy products for answers, according to a study conducted by Dr. Daniel Cramer of the Harvard Medical School. In the early 1990s, Dr. Cramer and his researchers found a link between milk and infertility.

The researchers discovered that women in Australia and Great Britain—countries where there is a high rate of milk consumption—had higher infertility rates, compared to women in Thailand, where very few dairy products are consumed. The Thai women, who generally are lactose intolerant, remain quite fertile well into their forties.

Researchers of the study concluded that high milk consumption among women, especially those thirty-five years and older may be harmful to human ova, and increase infertility rates. The scientists concluded that galactose—a simple sugar manufactured by the breakdown of lactose in all dairy milk—is toxic to ova. (Cheese, however, contains very small amounts of lactose, and has no apparent negative effects on conception.) It is, therefore, recommended that women who are trying to become pregnant reduce their milk consumption. During this period, they should substitute their diet with alternative sources of calcium from foods such as broccoli, oats, almonds, asparagus, lettuce, brewers yeast, and kelp.

Cottonseed Oil

A cotton byproduct, cottonseed oil *(Gossypium hirsutum)* has been used as a cooking oil in the United States. It is also used in many processed foods, such as mayonnaise and salad dressings, as well as commercial baked goods.

Since the 1970s, many studies, particularly those conducted in China, have indicated that men who regularly consume foods cooked in cottonseed oil suffer from decreased fertility due to lowered sperms counts. Gossypol, a component of cottonseeds, is toxic to sperm. In some extreme cases, the men have become permanently sterile.

The Brazilians have developed a contraceptive pill for men called Nofertil. Still in its testing stages, the pill, which contains gossypol, has been shown to suppress sperm production in men within two to three months of treatment. However, more safety and efficacy studies must be performed on Nofertil before it is made available to the public.

In addition to its effects on male fertility, cottonseed oil typically contains harmful pesticide residues, which have a toxic effect on the liver and gall bladder. It is also believed to irritate the digestive tract. Foods containing this oil should be avoided by everyone, even those who are not trying to conceive. Check food labels carefully.

SUMMING IT UP

Without creating undue panic, it is safe to say that prudent avoidance of the foods discussed in this chapter—soy products and other phytoestrogenic foods, peas, coffee, and products that contain cottonseed oil—can improve fertility in certain individuals. (Obviously, this applies only if there are no existing structural problems or infections.) While avoiding these foods is not necessarily a guarantee for becoming pregnant, it may certainly set the proper background for healthy eating, as further explained in the next chapter on vitamins and minerals.

5

Vitamins and Minerals

Vitamins and minerals play an integral role in maintaining one's overall health, including reproductive health. Unfortunately, the typical American diet is high in saturated fat, processed foods, and simple carbohydrates. It often lacks the vitamins, minerals, and amino acids that are necessary to maintain optimal health and well-being.

Our knowledge of the role of vitamins and minerals on the functioning of the human reproductive system is growing. Studies have shown that deficiencies in a number of certain nutrients can lead to fertility problems. This knowledge has given many fertility specialists cause to recommend that couples who are trying to conceive consume diets rich in vitamins A (beta-carotene), C, and E, the B-complex vitamins, essential fatty acids, and the minerals magnesium, selenium, and zinc. They also recommend the amino acids tyrosine for females and arginine and carnitine for males.

Each of these important nutrients for healthy reproduction is detailed in this chapter. Common food sources for each nutrient, as well as suggested supplemental recommendations are also offered. This information is summarized in Table 5.1 on page 76.

VITAMINS

Essential to life, vitamins contribute to good health mainly by assisting the processes that release energy from digested food. They are considered *micronutrients* because the body needs them in relatively small amounts compared with the four major nutrients—carbohydrates, fats, proteins, and water. Because they occur naturally in plants and animals, vitamins are considered organic.

Major vitamins are either fat-soluble or water-soluble. Water-soluble varieties, such as vitamin C and the B-complex vitamins, cannot be stored in the body and are excreted within one to four days. They need to be taken into the body daily. Fat-soluble vitamins, such as A, D, E, and K, can be stored for longer periods of time in the body's fatty tissue and the liver. For the body to function properly, it needs both water- and fat-soluble vitamins.

Cooking destroys valuable nutrients that are found in fruits and vegetables. Eating these foods in their raw state— or as close to their raw state as possible—is recommended.

Vitamin A (Beta-carotene)

A safe and effective immune system booster and antioxidant, vitamin A plays an important role in protecting the body from cancer and cardiovascular disease, and in maintaining healthy skin and proper eye function. Beta-carotene, a carotenoid that contains antioxidant properties, is converted to vitamin A in the body. Vitamin A and beta-carotene are also involved in maintaining healthy reproductive systems, including healthy ovarian functioning in women and healthy sperm in men.

One study indicated a link between low levels of beta-carotene, which is normally present in sperm, and *immuno-infertility*—infertility resulting from the presence of antibodies in sperm.

Food Sources: Vitamin A is found in fish liver oil, beef and chicken liver, eggs, and dairy products. Beta-carotene is present in green and yellow-orange fruits and vegetables such as carrots; kale; spinach, turnip, and beet greens; apricots; and cantaloupe.

Supplement Recommendation: For men, 10,000 international units of either vitamin A or beta-carotene daily is recommended. For women, 4,000 to 8,000 international units of beta-carotene daily is recommended.

* *Warning: High daily dosages of supplemental vitamin A (exceeding 10,000 international units) can be toxic to an unborn fetus and may result in birth defects. Therefore, pregnant women and women trying to conceive should avoid this supplement. On the other hand, beta-carotene, which is synthesized from vegetable sources, is safe.*

Vitamin B$_3$ (Niacin)

Vitamin B$_3$, or niacin, is essential for the production of sex hormones in both men and women.

Food Sources: Beef, pork, fish, milk and cheese, whole wheat products, potatoes, corn, eggs, dates, broccoli, tomatoes, and carrots.

Supplement Recommendation: Take at least 20 milligrams of niacin a day, which can be met by taking a 50-milligram B-complex vitamin.

Vitamin B$_5$ (Pantothenic Acid)

Known as the "anti-stress" vitamin, vitamin B$_5$ is essential for the production of estrogen and progesterone in women. A deficiency may cause impaired reproductive function.

Food Sources: Vitamin B₅ is found in beef, pork, saltwater fish, whole wheat and whole rye products, fresh broccoli, eggs, mushrooms, and cashews.

Supplement Recommendation: Take at least 10 milligrams of pantothenic acid daily, which can be met by taking a 50-milligram B-complex vitamin.

Vitamin B₆ (Pyridoxine)

Pyridoxine plays a role in reproductive gland function and in the proper balance of progesterone and estrogen levels. Several studies indicate a link between pyridoxine deficiency and insufficient progesterone production during the last part, or luteal phase, of the menstrual cycle. As seen in Chapter 1, progesterone is necessary for the building of the endometrial wall to house a fertilized egg.

In a 1979 study, fourteen women who had trouble conceiving due to low progesterone levels were given between 100 and 800 milligrams of supplemental B₆ daily. Within seven months of treatment, twelve of the women became pregnant.

Vitamin B₆ is also effective in reducing high levels of prolactin, a hormone released by the pituitary gland during pregnancy to stimulate the production of breast milk. Elevated levels of prolactin may cause ovulation to stop.

Food Sources: All foods contain small amounts of vitamin B₆; however, chicken, fish (especially herring and salmon), whole grains, wheat germ, eggs, bananas, spinach, carrots, sunflower seeds, walnuts, and avocados contain the highest amounts.

Supplement Recommendation: Take 100 milligrams of vitamin B₆ daily, along with a 50-milligram B-complex vitamin. Do not exceed 200 milligrams of vitamin B₆ without first consulting a doctor.

PABA (Para-Aminobenzoic Acid)

A nutrient often classified with the vitamin B-complex group, para-aminobenzoic acid (PABA) is a major component of folic acid. In addition to helping the body absorb vitamin B_5, PABA stimulates the pituitary gland to produce follicle-stimulating and luteinizing hormones. This may help encourage fertility in women who cannot conceive due to a reproductive hormonal imbalance. Those with liver disease and those with an alcohol dependency are likely to be deficient in PABA. The use of sulfa drugs, analgesics, and anticonvulsants may also cause a PABA deficiency.

Food Sources: Whole grains, mushrooms, spinach, oranges, eggs, molasses, and organ meats such as liver and kidneys are good sources of PABA.

Supplement Recommendation: Take 300 milligrams of PABA daily, particularly during the first half of the menstrual cycle. Do not take PABA if you are taking sulfa drugs.

Vitamin C

Men take note! Vitamin C is essential for healthy male reproductive function; a lack of this vitamin can result in low sperm counts. Research by Dr. Earl Dawson, an associate professor of obstetrics and gynecology at the University of Texas Medical School at Galveston, concluded that vitamin C plays a significant role in maintaining healthy sperm. Results of his studies showed that vitamin C deficiencies increase the risk of *sperm agglutination* (clumping). Dr. Dawson's studies also indicate that supplemental vitamin C improves sperm count, motility, and vitality, particularly in men who smoke.

Food Sources: Berries, citrus fruits, and green vegetables are excellent sources of vitamin C. Good sources include asparagus, avocados, beet and turnip greens, Brussels sprouts, cabbage, grapefruit, papaya, pineapple, strawberries, spinach,

Dandelion Greens—
The Liver Cleanser

The common dandelion—every gardener's nemesis—has been used for medicinal purposes throughout the world for hundreds of years. Its bitter green leaves help purify the blood, detoxify the liver, and cleanse the kidneys. What does this have to do with optimum fertility? The liver, in particular, is important for helping maintain healthy reproductive function.

In addition to its important role in digestion and energy production, the liver acts as a detoxifier. It combines toxic substances—metabolic waste, drugs, alcohol, and other harmful chemicals—with less toxic substances, then excretes them through the kidneys. In this capacity, it also breaks down excess amounts of estrogen. However, if the liver is overworked, as can happen when it is burdened, for instance, under the strain of fatty and/or processed foods, alcohol, or medications, its detoxifying ability can be compromised. Among other results, reproductive function can be negatively affected by the accumulation of excess estrogen.

A properly functioning liver is critical for good health, which is why proper dietary nutrition is so important. Rich in vitamins A, C, and E, as well as B vitamins and the mineral zinc, dandelion greens are excellent for cleansing the liver. Its leaves can be juiced or tossed into a salad and eaten fresh. Dandelion greens are quite bitter; however, light steaming will help remove this bitterness. They are also available in capsule form and are sold in most health food stores.

When purchasing fresh dandelion greens, try to choose only those which have been organically grown without the use of chemical fertilizers or pesticides. Many grocery stores and produce markets carry this organic type.

tomatoes, and sweet peppers.

Supplement Recommendation: For increased sperm health in men, take 1,000 milligrams of vitamin C daily. (In Dr. Dawson's study, the greatest improvement was seen in those men who stayed on this regimen for at least one month.)

Vitamin E

Vitamin E is an antioxidant that is beneficial in its ability to neutralize dangerous free radicals. It is also important in maintaining healthy male and female reproductive systems. In women, vitamin E can help alleviate some of the symptoms associated with premenstrual syndrome (PMS), while deficiencies have been implicated in miscarriage and uterine degeneration. In men, vitamin E's antioxidizing capability is believed to be responsible for protecting sperm against cellular damage.

One three-month study conducted in Israel, involved fifteen men whose partners were undergoing *in vitro* fertilization. The men displayed low fertilization rates. In other words, even though the men had normal sperm, the sperm had not been able to fertilize their partners' eggs. During the course of the study, the men were given a daily 200-milligram dosage of vitamin E. After a period of only one month, the fertilization rates increased dramatically.

Food Sources: Particularly rich sources of vitamin E are found in the fats contained in vegetables. Unprocessed vegetable oils, such as cottonseed, corn, olive, soybean, safflower, and wheat germ, have the highest concentrations. Green leafy vegetables, apples, mangos, nuts, eggs, and oatmeal are other good sources.

Supplement Recommendation: Take 400 to 800 international units of vitamin E daily.

* ***Warning:*** *Vitamin E is a blood thinner. Those taking anti-coagu-*

lants or those who experience prolonged bleeding time should consult a physician or nutritionist before taking vitamin E supplements.

ESSENTIAL FATTY ACIDS

Sometimes referred to as vitamin F, or "good" fats, essential fatty acids (EFAs) are necessary for optimal health. Unable to be produced by the body, EFAs must be acquired through food or supplements. They must not be subjected to heat, either in processing or cooking. Omega 3 and omega 6 are the two basic categories of essential fatty acids. Both types are necessary for maintaining healthy reproductive systems. For instance, EFAs are effective in normalizing cervical mucus that is too thick for sperm to move through.

Omega-3 Fatty Acids

The omega-3 family of EFAs includes alpha-linolenic acid, eicosapentaenoic acid (EPA), and docosahexaenoic acid (DHA). These fats can help reduce cholesterol, improve brain function, and help alleviate the pain of arthritis. In addition, these fats appear to improve the function of the glandular system. Women with high levels of estrogen may benefit from omega 3 as it is an estrogen blocker. It reduces excessive amounts of estrogen produced by the ovaries, and may increase follicle-stimulating hormone levels, much like the fertility drug Clomid.

Food Sources: Salmon, bluefin tuna, mackerel, herring, sardines and oils from these fish are rich sources of omega-3 oils. Other excellent sources include dark green leafy vegetables and canola, flaxseed, and walnut oils

Supplement Recommendation: Flaxseed oil capsules may be taken to supplement food sources, especially for those who are not big fish eaters. Flaxseed oil is nontoxic and should be taken according to label directions.

Omega-6 Fatty Acids

Omega-6 EFAs include linoleic and gamma-linoleic acids. Along with omega-3 EFAs, omega-6 oils help regulate hormonal balance. They do this by increasing estrogen levels in the body. If low estrogen levels are the reason for infertility, omega 6 may be helpful.

Food Sources: Unsaturated vegetable oils, such as canola, primrose, sesame, and soybean are excellent sources. Good sources include raw nuts, seeds, and legumes.

Supplement Recommendation: Omega-6 fatty acids are best consumed through food sources; however, a 500-milliliter capsule of evening primrose oil twice a day can be taken as a supplement.

MINERALS

Essential in nerve responses, muscle contractions, and the internal processing of nutrients, minerals are also important for forming bones and blood, and for maintaining proper metabolism and a healthy immune system. Minerals fall into two categories—bulk and trace. Bulk minerals include calcium, magnesium, sodium, potassium, and phosphorus, and are needed in larger amounts than trace minerals. Although trace minerals, such as chromium, iron, selenium, sulfur, and zinc, are required in minute amounts, they are still necessary for good health. Three minerals that are particularly important for good reproductive health include magnesium, selenium, and zinc.

Magnesium

A bulk mineral, magnesium works with dozens of different enzymes that facilitate processes throughout the body, including the metabolism of protein, fat, and carbohydrates. It is also necessary for the proper functioning of the reproductive system.

A 1994 study at the Biolab Medical Unit in London, England, included a group of women with low red blood cell magnesium (RBC-Mg) levels who were experiencing difficulty in conceiving for no apparent reason. During the course of the study, all of the women were given magnesium supplements. Within eight months, all of the women conceived and subsequently gave birth to healthy babies.

Food Sources: The largest quantities of magnesium are found in dairy products, fish, meat, apples, wheat, brown rice, bananas, and tofu.

Supplement Recommendation: Take 600 milligrams of magnesium daily.

Selenium

Although the trace mineral selenium is present in all tissues of the body, it is concentrated mostly in the kidneys, liver, spleen, pancreas, and testes. Selenium's most important role in the body is as an antioxidant; however, it is also an important component of sperm, significantly improving its motility. Deficiencies have been linked to infertility in men. The connection between selenium and female infertility is not as clear.

Food Sources: Richest sources of selenium include seafood, meats, brown rice, soybeans, and whole grains. Although fruits and vegetables typically contain very low amounts of selenium, beets, bell peppers, and leafy green vegetables contain some.

Supplement Recommendation: For those who do not consume selenium-rich foods regularly, take 60 to 100 micrograms of selenium daily along with 400 international units of vitamin E.

Zinc

Critical for the synthesis of RNA and DNA, which are essential for cell division, zinc is also important in the production of testosterone. Low zinc levels also may result in reduced sperm counts and poor sperm motility. Several studies have also linked zinc deficiencies in females to miscarriage and complications during pregnancy.

Food Sources: Although zinc is present in nearly all foods, it is especially plentiful in fish and other seafood (particularly oysters), meats, poultry (especially dark meat), liver, eggs, legumes, mushrooms, pumpkin and sunflower seeds, soybeans, and whole grains.

Royal Jelly

Royal jelly, so named because it was coveted by British royalty for its nutritional value, is a vitamin- and protein-rich substance produced by worker bees (specifically a special group of nurse bees) and fed to the queen bee of the colony.

Taking royal jelly is akin to taking a megavitamin. Most of the vitamins necessary for proper reproductive function are found in royal jelly. The substance contains all of the B-complex vitamins, as well as twenty-two amino acids, magnesium, zinc, and antibacterial and antibiotic components. It is also rich in the nucleic acids RNA and DNA—the very stuff from which life is made.

Royal jelly has long been credited with rejuvenating and regenerating properties; it has also been connected to renewed sexual power. Most effective in liquid form, which comes in vials, royal jelly is sold in health food stores and is safe to drink daily. It is also sold in capsules.

Supplement Recommendation: Take up to 50 milligrams of zinc daily.

* Warning: Do not take more than 50 milligrams of zinc per day. Higher doses can impair immune function and deplete copper levels.

AMINO ACIDS

Amino acids are organic chemical compounds that form the building blocks of proteins, a necessary part of every living

Table 5.1. Foods for Healthy Reproductive Function

The following foods are rich in many of the nutrients necessary for good health and proper reproductive function.

	Vitamin A	Vitamin B_3	Vitamin B_5	Vitamin B_6	Vitamin C
Bananas				♥	♥
Beans			♥	♥	
Cantaloupes	♥	♥		♥	♥
Carrots	♥	♥		♥	♥
Eggs				♥	
Garlic				♥	
Leafy greens	♥				
Nuts					
Oranges					
Poultry				♥	
Pumpkin	♥				♥
Salmon		♥			
Tuna		♥		♥	
Vegetable oils					
Whole wheat products			♥		

cell in the body. Protein makes up the building blocks of muscles, bones, blood, glands, hormones, hair, nails, and internal organs. Amino acids also enable vitamins and minerals to perform their jobs properly. Our liver produces about 80 percent of the amino acids that we need; these are considered *nonessential*. The remaining 20 percent must be obtained through diet and are considered *essential amino acids*. Tyrosine, arginine, and carnitine are especially important for reproductive health.

Vitamin E (essential fatty acids)	Vitamin F	PABA	Selenium	Magnesium	Zinc
				♥	
♥					
				♥	
		♥		♥	
			♥		
♥				♥	
♥	♥			♥	
♥					
			♥		♥
				♥	
	♥		♥	♥	
♥	♥				♥
♥		♥	♥	♥	♥

Tyrosine

The amino acid tyrosine is helpful in regulating the pituitary gland and maintaining the proper balance between estrogen and progesterone levels.

Food Sources: Almonds, avocados, bananas, dairy products, lima beans, and pumpkin and sesame seeds are good sources of tyrosine.

Supplement Recommendation: Take up to 500 milligrams of supplemental tyrosine daily.

* Warning: Those taking monoamine oxidase (MAO) inhibitors— commonly prescribed for depression—should limit their intake of foods containing tyrosine, and should not take any supplemental l-tyrosine. This can lead to a sudden and dangerous rise in blood pressure.

Carnitine

Although carnitine is actually a substance related to the B vitamins, its chemical structure is so similar to that of amino acids, it is usually considered together with them. Unlike true amino acids, carnitine is not used for protein synthesis. Instead, it increases the use of fat as an energy source, preventing fatty buildups, especially in the heart, liver, and muscles. Studies have also shown that supplemental carnitine can increase the quality of sperm.

The body can manufacture carnitine as long as sufficient amounts of vitamins B_1, B_6, and C are present. However, those who typically do not consume proper amounts of protein, or those who are unable to digest food properly, can have a carnitine deficiency.

Food Sources: Rich sources of carnitine include fish, eggs, and other foods of animal origin.

Supplement Recommendation: Men should take 3 grams of supplemental carnitine daily.

Arginine

A nonessential amino acid manufactured in the body, arginine is important in the production of sperm (80 percent of semen is composed of arginine). Supplemental arginine can help increase sperm count and improve sperm quality.

Supplement Recommendation: Men should take 1,500 milligrams of supplemental arginine daily.

* *Warning: Individuals with herpes should not take arginine supplements as it can stimulate an outbreak of the virus.*

SUMMING IT UP

Eating wisely is the key to maintaining optimal health and preventing infertility that is related to a nutrient deficiency. Eating a well-balanced diet that is rich in grains, fish, and fresh fruits and vegetables is highly recommended. Limit your intake of saturated and hydrogenated fats, which are found in butter, margarine, and fried and creamy foods. Instead of margarine, use omega-rich vegetable oils such as canola or soy. If your diet is lacking certain nutrients, make an effort to eat more nutrient-rich foods and take the proper supplements. Vitamin and mineral supplements should not replace a healthy diet. Remember, a proper diet combined with a stress-free lifestyle and clean living environment are important factors in helping to overcome infertility naturally.

6

Herbal and Homeopathic Treatments

No one can argue that modern medicine has presented tremendous cures for a great number of illnesses and medical conditions. Medications, immunizations, diagnostic tools, and modern surgical procedures have been instrumental in saving or improving the lives of many. Such medical strides, however, have come with a downside. With so much focus on curing illness with drugs and synthetic compounds that are formulated in laboratories, the use of natural remedies such as herbals and homeopathic preparations has taken a back seat. There has also been less focus on the actual prevention of certain illnesses.

In most cases, laboratory-produced medications are very powerful in their healing abilities, but are not necessarily more effective than herbal remedies. Furthermore, their likelihood of causing side effects is greater. Interestingly, many modern-day medicines are based on plant remedies. Acetylsalicylic acid found in aspirin, for example, originally was derived from the white willow plant.

Since the 1990s, there has been a renewed interest in

herbal remedies. This is due, partly because of the number of known side effects of conventional medicines, and partly because of the growing public awareness of the effectiveness of herbs and other natural remedies. This chapter takes a look at some of the herbs that were used by the ancient Chinese, Greeks, and North American Indians to boost reproductive function. It also presents the plant-derived homeopathic remedies that have been used since the 1800s.

HERBS

For centuries, the medicinal benefits of herbs have been known by almost every culture in the world. Many herbs contain ingredients that, when used correctly, can help heal the body. Other herbs are effectively used as preventives.

A woman's ability to conceive is a reflection not only of the health of her reproductive system but ultimately the health of her entire mind, body, and spirit. Certain herbs, along with proper nutrition, regular exercise, and an overall healthy lifestyle and living environment can assist in harmonizing the body's natural order. More specifically, a number of herbs can be particularly helpful for women who experience trouble conceiving due to hormonal imbalance. By stimulating the pituitary glands and ovaries, certain herbs cause the production and balance of luteinizing hormone (LH), follicle-stimulating hormone (FSH), estrogen, and progesterone in women. Certain herbs also encourage the proper balance of testosterone in men. Obviously, there are certain physiological causes of infertility that cannot be reversed by herbs, but for those women who have trouble conceiving due to hormone imbalance, herbal treatments may prove to be quite effective.

Five herbs in particular—chaste tree, false unicorn root, red raspberry leaves, dong quai, and licorice root—are commonly recommended for treating infertility in women. When beginning an herbal regimen, patience is crucial. Some individuals may experience benefits within one to two months, while others may take longer.

Note that the active ingredients in herbs are most potent when they are freshly picked. However, if the herbs are thoroughly dried, they can retain their medicinal value for years. The fresh leaves, bark, and roots of herbs can be used in their natural form, or in tablets, capsules, powders, extracts or tinctures, and oils. The leaves, bark, berries, seeds, roots, and flowers are also available in their dried form.

Ground herbal powder can be purchased loose or in capsule form. Loose leaves, flowers, or other delicate parts of herbs are often steeped, not boiled, in hot water and taken as a tea. Extracts are made by crushing the herbs through a press, then soaking them in alcohol or water. Tinctures are similar to extracts, except the herbs are soaked in water only—not alcohol. The excess water or alcohol evaporates, leaving a concentrated extract, which is very potent. Essential oils are derived from herbs through steam distillation or cold pressing. They are usually mixed with water or oil and used as a mouthwash, eyewash, inhalant, or douche. These oils are also used externally on cuts and burns. Essential oils should be diluted before being applied to the body, and they should not be taken internally unless instructed by a qualified health care professional. (More on essential oils in Chapter 7, "Flower Power.")

While the herbs listed in this chapter are considered safe, it is important to keep in mind that herbs in general are powerful medicine. An herbal preparation that is beneficial to one person may cause an allergic reaction in someone else. And combinations of certain herbs can also produce negative side effects. For this reason, it is strongly suggested that you consult an herbalist, naturopathic doctor, or other qualified health-care provider who is well-versed on herbal remedies before starting any regimen.

The following herbs, which have found to be effective for treating infertility, are summarized in Table 6.1 on page 87.

Chaste Tree (*Vitex agnus-castus*)

Chaste tree, also called chasteberry, is one of the most impor-tant herbs used to treat infertility caused by hormonal imbal-ance. Its acts on the pituitary gland to stimulate the release of luteinizing hormone (LH) and to mildly inhibit excess folli-cle-stimulating hormone (FSH). It also helps restore proper estrogen and progesterone balance, while preventing high prolactin levels—inhibitors of ovulation.

Chaste tree is also recommended if the cause of infertility is due to fibroids or a corpus luteum abnormality such as luteal phase defect. This herb stimulates the corpus luteum to produce adequate amounts of estrogen and progesterone to help build the endometrial wall and lengthen the luteal phase in those women whose periods are abnormally short. It is also indicated for irregular, scanty, or painful menstruation, as well as premenstrual syndrome and other disorders related to hormonal function. After the use of birth control pills, chaste tree may be of value in helping the reproductive system regain its natural balance. Because of its hormonal effects, chaste tree may be effective in cases of ovarian cysts and endometriosis.

After taking chaste tree for only two menstrual cycles, some women begin to experience its positive effects. For oth-ers, chaste tree may take up to seven months before showing signs of effectiveness.

Recommendations: Unless otherwise instructed, take 10 to 15 drops of chaste tree extract three times a day, from day ten of the menstrual cycle through the first day of the following cycle. To lessen the bitterness of the drops, take them in a small amount of water. Chaste tree's effectiveness should be seen within seven or eight months. If there are no results within this time period, discontinue its use.

* *Warning: Do not take chaste tree without first discussing it with a doctor of naturopathic medicine. Chaste tree must be used with*

caution. It has been linked to the release of multiple eggs and may, therefore, result in multiple births. Also, as chaste tree is a suppressor of the male hormone testosterone, men whose partners are trying to conceive should not take it. Animal studies have indicated that this herb can slow or even stop sperm production.

False Unicorn Root (*Chamaelirium luteum*)

False unicorn root, also called helonias, is an herb native to North America. Considered one of the best herbs for strengthening the reproductive system, false unicorn root is commonly used by herbalists to treat female infertility. It helps strengthen the endometrial wall and encourages follicular growth in the ovaries. False unicorn root is particularly helpful for women with low levels of follicle-stimulating hormone, and those women who experience luteal phase defect. This herb is also helpful in preventing miscarriage.

Recommendations: Unless instructed otherwise, take 7 to 15 drops of false unicorn extract three times daily, from day seven of the menstrual cycle through the first day of the following cycle. This regimen is recommended for up to five months.

Red Raspberry Leaves (*Rubus idaeus*)

The leaves of the red raspberry plant, also known as garden raspberry, are excellent in strengthening the entire reproductive system. Specifically, red raspberry is helpful in toning the uterine muscles, preparing them for conception and pregnancy.

Recommendations: Unless otherwise instructed, take 10 drops of red raspberry extract up to three times daily, from day seven of the menstrual cycle through the first day of the following cycle for five months.

Dong Quai *(Radix angelica sinensis)*

Considered the "queen of herbs," dong quai, also called Chinese angelica, is a small plant that resembles parsley. It is the root of this plant, however, that contains most of its medicinal qualities. Dong quai, which should be taken after ovulation, helps to balance and stimulate hormones, especially progesterone, which is important in strengthening the uterine wall for conception. It is most beneficial in women with short periods or luteal phase defect.

The male reproductive system is also aided by dong quai. Ferulic acid, one of this herb's chemicals, helps increase the motility and viability of sperm.

Recommendations: Unless instructed otherwise, take 10 to 15 drops of dong quai extract twice daily, from day fourteen (or the estimated day of ovulation) through the first day of the next menstrual cycle, for five months. As the quality of dong quai capsules vary (some brands contain up to 85 percent millet as filler), extract is the recommended form. Dong quai is particularly effective when taken with red raspberry leaves.

Licorice Root *(Glycyrrhiza glabra)*

Licorice root is a phytoestrogen—a plant containing estrogenic properties. It can be helpful for those women who are *amenorrheac* (without menstrual cycles due to a dysfunction of either the hypothalamus or pituitary glands), or those who have short menstrual cycles (under twenty-four days) on a continual basis. Taking licorice root may help normalize low estrogen levels, and, therefore, menstrual cycles.

Recommendations: Unless instructed otherwise, take 10 drops of licorice root extract twice daily, from day ten through day thirteen of the menstrual cycle for three months.

* *Warning:* Licorice root should not be used during pregnancy, or by those with diabetes, glaucoma, heart disease, or high

Table 6.1. Helpful Herbs for Fertility

The following is a list of conditions associated with infertility, and the herbs most beneficial in treating them. The days on which it is best to take these herbs is also included. For most individuals, the herbs mentioned below can be safely taken together.

Always check with a qualified health-care professional, such as an herbalist or naturopath, before taking any herbal regimen. In most instances, however, following package directions is appropriate.

Condition	Helpful Herbs	Day of Cycle to Begin Regimen*
Short menstrual cycles lasting less than 24 days (luteal phase defect)	• Chaste tree extract	10
	• Dong quai extract	14
	• Red raspberry tea or extract	7
	• False unicorn root extract	7
Short, scanty menstrual periods—lasting 1 to 3 days	• Licorice root extract	10 (for no more than 4 days)
	• False unicorn root extract	7
Fibroids	• Chaste tree extract	10
	• False unicorn root extract	7
High prolactin levels	• Chaste tree extract	10
Long and irregular menstrual periods; menstrual cycles lasting more than 33 days	• Chaste tree extract	10
	• False unicorn root extract	7
	• Red raspberry tea or extract	7
Polycystic ovaries (High luteinizing hormone levels, low progesterone levels)	• False unicorn root extract	7
	• Dong quai extract	14
	• Red raspberry tea or extract	7
Tendency to miscarry (due to low progesterone levels)	• False unicorn root extract	7
	• Dong quai extract	14
	• Red raspberry tea or extract	7

*Unless otherwise specified, continue taking herbs until beginning of the next cycle.

blood pressure. As it promotes the conversion of testosterone into estrogen, licorice should be avoided by anyone with an estrogen-sensitive disorder, such as fibrocystic breasts or polycystic ovaries. Women with endometriosis should avoid licorice as well. It should not be used on a daily basis for more than seven days in a row, as it can result in high blood pressure in those with previously normal blood pressure.

HOMEOPATHIC TREATMENTS

Homeopathy is a system of healing developed in Germany by Dr. Samuel Hahnemann in the early 1800s. His research in this field began when he discovered that minute dilutions of natural substances from plants, minerals, and animals could cause certain physical and emotional disease-like symptoms in humans. However, when these same weakened substances were given to patients already suffering from the very conditions that the substances were known to cause, the symptoms disappeared, and the patients became well again.

When it comes to medicine, the traditional notion has always been that the higher the dosage, the greater its effect. In homeopathic medicine, just the opposite is true. Odd as it may seem, the more a homeopathic substance is diluted, the greater its potency. Hahnemann concluded that these diluted substances (which he later formulated into "homeopathic" remedies) could target specific symptoms of an illness by stimulating the body's natural healing response to cure them. This led Hahnemann to the observation that "like cures like." In other words, a substance that in large doses produces the symptoms of an illness, in very minute doses, actually cures it. This phenomenon is called the Law of Similars.

The conventional medical establishment has often questioned the authenticity of homeopathy, whose principles seem to be completely opposite to those of traditional medicine. Probably one of the biggest differences lies in the dosage size of prescribed treatments. Homeopathic medicine is prescribed in minute doses, the power of which is believed to come from *vibratory energy*. In physics, vibratory energy is a means of storing energy. All matter, be it solid, liquid, or gas, can store energy in its molecules, and re-radiate it at a later time. Therefore, when a mineral, plant, or animal substance is placed in water and shaken, the water molecules absorb the vibratory energy of the material substance, and thus, its healing abilities.

Those who practice homeopathy believe it is a healing process that not only alleviates symptoms, but also re-establishes the body's internal order—physical, mental, and emotional. This school of medicine has enjoyed much support in Europe since the late 1800s. Recently, it has seen a rise in popularity in the United States as well.

When homeopaths prescribe remedies to women with infertility problems, they focus not only on physical symptoms but on emotional symptoms as well. A homeopath considers the entire "constitutional state" of the patient. For instance, an infertility patient might display physical signs that include heavy menstrual bleeding, tender breasts, and scant or irregular periods. Emotional signs may include depression, fear, and anxiety. According to the patient's symptoms, the homeopath will prescribe a number of remedies that are known to induce these exact conditions (or symptoms). Generally, homeopaths will prescribe a certain dosage for two to three weeks, at which point, the symptoms should begin to subside and then disappear.

It is imperative that a professional homeopath or naturopath be consulted prior to taking homeopathic treatments. To begin with, proper diagnosis is important. Plus, there are many different homeopathic remedies that can be used to treat infertility, and only a trained specialist can determine the most appropriate types for an individual's particular needs. A specialist is also necessary for determining proper dosages.

The following homeopathic remedies have been effective in treating the causes of many types of female infertility, including, but not limited to, hormone imbalances, stress, anxiety, and even unexplained infertility (infertility that has no medical explanation).

The physical symptoms that a homeopath looks for prior to prescribing remedies for infertile patients include irregular periods, frequent miscarriages, cramping, and heavy bleeding. Homeopaths also consider such conditions as fatigue, depression, lethargy, and anxiety in determining which homeopathic remedy is best suited for the patient.

- *Conium macultum* is particularly recommended for women who need to get in touch with their feelings. On a physical level, Conium may be particularly beneficial for women with scanty periods and painful breasts—the result of high prolactin levels.

- *Apis mellifera* is generally recommended for women who are dealing with anxiety and "pent up" emotions, and experiencing physical symptoms such as very heavy periods and painful ovaries.

- *Cantharis* is generally recommended for treating vaginal itching, heavy periods, and excessive vaginal discharge. (Vaginal itching may be caused by a sexually transmitted disease or a candida infection. Women with severe vaginal itching should consult a physician for a full diagnosis.)

There are many more homeopathic remedies suitable for varying symptoms, and a trained specialist can determine which remedy is the most appropriate for you. For further information on homeopathic treatments for infertility, the following books are excellent resources: *Homeopathy for Women: A Comprehensive, Easy-to-Use Guide for Women of All Ages* by Barry Rose and Christina Scott-Moncrieff (North Pomfret, VT: Trafalgar Square Publishing, 1998), and *Complete Guide to Homeopathy* by Andrew Lockie and Nicola Geddes (DK Publishing, 1995).

SUMMING IT UP

Herbal and homeopathic remedies have truly marvelous healing potential, and the ones listed in this chapter are particularly suitable for restoring the natural balance of the reproductive system. Both types of remedies can be effective when used alone; however, when they are combined with other forms of therapy, such as meditation, flower essences, or massage, their effects are enhanced even further. In the next chapter, you will learn more about the healing power of one of these forms—plant essences.

7

Flower Power

Flower essences and aromatic essential oils (also called volatile oils), which have been used by many cultures for thousands of years, are both derived from plants. Every plant has its own special qualities and properties, many of which can be used for healing. Typically, these plant remedies do not target the actual symptoms of a condition the way pharmaceutical medications do. Rather, they address the underlying mental or emotional imbalances caused by blocked energy channels within the body. It is believed that when these channels are blocked, illness can set in. Treating underlying causes, rather than symptoms alone is a whole body approach to dealing with health conditions.

Research has shown that essential oils and flower essences can influence a person's emotional state by reducing stress levels, easing feelings of depression, and creating a sense of calm and tranquility. Each plant species is believed to be in tune with a different human emotion, and each possesses the ability to alleviate negative emotions such as fear, anxiety, and hopelessness. Like homeopathic treatments, these plant remedies are believed to contain infinitesimal amounts of the material substance from which they are made. It is not, however, the actual physical properties of the plants that give them their healing ability, but rather the healing energy of the plants themselves.

Typically, illnesses or conditions, including infertility, that are entirely physiological in nature and unrelated to one's emotional state are not successfully treated with plant essences. However, because many researchers have linked stress and anxiety to hormonal imbalances, plant extracts have long been used by women whose infertility may be caused by such an imbalance. In combination with stress-management techniques such as meditation, plant essences may be effective in helping rebalance emotional states and encourage conception in certain cases.

AROMATHERAPY AND ESSENTIAL OILS

Aromatherapy is the practice of using essential oils to stimulate positive changes in the body. Essential oils are highly concentrated, scented, non-oily essences derived from the flowers, leaves, and other parts of certain plants. These oils are stored in a plant's cells, and, according to botanists, control a number of plant functions, including cellular metabolism and photosynthesis. Not all plants, however, produce essential oils. In fact, only a few hundred of the thousands of plant species on earth do. Essential oils are extracted through steaming or cold-pressing.

Like herbs, essential oils have been used by various civilizations for thousands of years to maintain general well-being, prevent disease, and promote healing. Over 3,000 years ago, Egyptian priests used aromatic oils to treat depression and anxiety. Hippocrates, the ancient Greek founder of Western medicine, recommended aromatic essential oils for maintaining general good health.

Aromatic oils have been used for centuries as inhalants in

baths, massage oils, and compresses. Today you can find them in candles and air fresheners as well. Essential oils are not to be taken internally, as they can cause a toxic reaction.

When inhaled, aromatic oils stimulate the olfactory nerves, which relay information to the limbic system in the brain. This system is responsible for a number of activities, including memory, learning, and emotions. The hypothalamus, which is part of the limbic system, is responsible for coordinating the production of reproductive hormones within the pituitary gland. It also controls the production of endorphin hormones necessary for maintaining stress levels. Essential oils gently alter mood and restore energy. For this reason, they are believed to be influential in balancing the body at the emotional level, which, in turn, affects the physical level.

When used for massage, the active constituents contained in the oils are absorbed through the pores and into the bloodstream. These oils should not, however, be applied directly to the skin. They are so concentrated and so potent that they may irritate or even burn the skin. Before using essential oils for massage, they must be diluted properly with a carrier oil. Generally, carrier oils are extracted from nuts and seeds, although some vegetable oils are acceptable. Unscented, cold-pressed oils, such as almond, canola, grapeseed, sunflower, and jojoba are the ones most commonly used. Carrier oils also enable an essential oil to be spread more evenly and easily over the skin. They are also economical—less essential oil is needed to cover a greater area of skin.

Pure essential oils can be purchased in special aromatherapy stores as well as some health food stores. Not all essential oils, however, are the same. They come in a wide range of qualities, which are often reflected in the price. Be aware—inexpensive brands are likely to be inferior. Always look for the words "essential oil" on the label. Many so-called essential oils are labeled as "aromatherapy oil," "pure botanical fragrance," "essential oil blend," or "botanical perfume." To help assure that you are getting pure essential oil, the product label should say "pure essential oil" and nothing else. Instructions for use should be followed according to label directions. And always purchase essential oils that come in brown-tinted glass bottles, which help block light from spoiling the contents.

A few aromatic essential oils are commonly recommended by aromatherapists for treating infertility. Some are helpful for women, others are helpful for men, and some are helpful for both. The most popular of these oils are presented in the following discussions.

Rose Oil

There are approximately 5,000 species of roses, but basically only two—the damask rose and the cabbage rose—are used to produce essential oil for aromatherapy. Because such a large quantity of roses (approximately 60,000) are required to distill only one ounce of rose oil, it is fairly expensive. It does, however, have significant therapeutic value.

Used for thousands of years by various civilizations, including the ancient Egyptians and Greeks, rose oil has known anti-inflammatory and antimicrobial agents. It is also considered effective in balancing estrogen and progesterone levels, making it a good choice for women who are experiencing infertility due to hormonal imbalance, fibroid tumors, or endometriosis. Rose oil is also considered effective in increasing sexual desire and reducing stress, tension, and anxiety. Therefore sexual issues such as frigidity and impotence that are stress-related, also respond positively to rose oil.

Geranium oil

Geranium oil is extracted from only a few of the many hundreds of geranium flower species. The entire plant is steam-distilled to produce this essential oil.

Among its many uses, geranium oil is believed to balance hormones by stimulating the adrenal cortex. This organ secretes androgen hormones, which are the precursors of testosterone and estrogen. Geranium oil is recommended for both women and men in helping to create the right hormonal balance to encourage fertility.

* **Warning:** *Those with hypoglycemia (low blood sugar) should avoid geranium oil, as it can lower blood sugar levels.*

Jasmine Oil

Fragrant jasmine flowers are native to China, India, and the Mediterranean. Approximately 1,000 pounds of these flowers are needed to produce only one pound of essential oil.

Ideal for its calming, relaxing effects, jasmine is also helpful as a hormone balancer. It is also believed to strengthen the male reproductive system, and has been used traditionally by Japanese men who have reproductive problems.

Melissa Oil

Also known as lemon balm oil, melissa oil has many positive benefits for women. It is considered a good uterine tonic, and can help regulate menstrual cycles and heavy menstrual bleeding. Melissa oil also helps ease emotional tension and can encourage a general calming effect.

FLOWER ESSENCES

Flower essences are odorless liquid plant extracts. While herbal extracts and essential oils contain large amounts of the physical properties of the plant from which they originate, flower essences contain the vibrational (healing) energy of the plant. They are believed to restore emotional well-being to the body by unblocking negative emotions and behavior patterns that can cause physical illness. Like essential oils,

Fertility Massage Blend

A massage using the following combination of essential oils is suggested to help promote fertility. Gently work the blend into the pelvic area as well as the nape of the neck.

10 drops rose oil

5 drops jasmine oil

5 drops geranium oil

3 drops melissa oil

30 milliliters (2 tablespoons) of a carrier oil, such as almond or jojoba

flower remedies specifically address a person's emotional state, creating mental balance. This, in turn, facilitates psychological as well as physiological well-being.

A woman's emotional state can influence her reproduction system. Feelings of stress and anxiety as well as guilt, despair, fear, and anger can cause an imbalance in reproductive hormones and prevent ovulation. Many women as well as men who have experienced difficulty conceiving due to emotional discord have found flower essences to be helpful.

Flower essences have been used for thousands of years for their healing abilities; however, it was not until the 1930s that they were studied intensively by Dr. Edward Bach, a Welsh physician and homeopath. Dr. Bach theorized that the cause of disease and illness originated in part from a person's negative emotions. He further theorized that these emotions could lower a person's resistance to disease and illness. Therefore, if the emotional condition is treated, illness would fade.

Bach developed thirty-eight plant essences, each one corresponding to a negative emotional state. He claimed that each of the essences contained the vibrational energy of the plant from which it was derived and could rebalance a par-

ticular negative emotional state. In addition to Bach's remedies, there are many other flower essences available.

In order to obtain the flower's vibrational energy, typically essences are prepared by placing fresh-picked flowers in a
bowl of spring water, then setting the bowl in the sunlight for
three to five hours. The flowers' healing energy is released
into the water. Flowers that are picked in the early morning
when their blooms are full and filled with dew are the best.
After the flowers are removed from the bowl, the flower
water is poured halfway into a sterilized bottle. Brandy is
poured into the remaining half of the bottle. This concentra-
tion is called the "mother essence" or "mother tincture," and
can be used as is or in dilutions.

Because flower essences work at the psychological level to
balance emotions, it is necessary to correctly determine the
specific negative emotional conditions that exist. (If the
wrong flower essence is taken, however, it will not produce
negative side effects. The essence simply won't correct the
emotional condition.) Finding the right flower essence is not
always easy, so consulting with a naturopath who possesses a
knowledge of flower remedies is recommended.

Flower essences should be taken when one is most
relaxed—perhaps before going to bed, when meditating, or
while practicing some other form of relaxation. Simply place
5 to 10 drops of the essence under the tongue, twice a day for
two to four weeks. If there is no change in the emotional state
after four weeks, stop taking the essence for two weeks, then
repeat the process again. If there is still no change, the flower
essence is most likely not the correct one for your condition.

Of the many flower essences that have been used effectively for treating infertility, gorse, lady's mantle, olive, pine,
and she oak flower essences are the most popular. They can
be helpful in balancing negative emotions, particularly stress
and anxiety, that may be underlying links to infertility.

While most flower essences, especially the Bach flower
remedies, are readily available in health food stores, others

may be a little more difficult to come by. If you have trouble finding a particular essence, try contacting one of the following mail order companies:

Flower Vision Research
PO Box 43627
Upper Montclair, NJ 07043
(800) 298–4434
(973) 746–5798
(973) 746–4321 (FAX)
email:
  essences@flowervr.com
website:
  www.flowervr.com

Flower Essence Pharmacy
PO Box 1147
Sandy, OR 97055
(800) 343–8693
(503) 668–7160
(503) 862–1408 (FAX)
email:
  info@floweressences.com
website:
  www.floweressences.com

Gorse Flower Essence

Gorse is a Bach flower essence that is typically recommended for those who feel a sense of hopelessness and loss of certainty—those who generally are afraid of change and the unknown. Gorse flower essence helps adjust these negative mindsets, allowing the individual to see things more positively and develop a sense of faith and hope.

Lady's Mantle Essence

Lady's mantle essence, derived from the *Alchemilla vulgaris* flower, is recommended to help balance negative emotions that are related to female sexuality and pregnancy. Women who have deep-rooted fears of pregnancy, labor, and/or delivery may find this flower remedy helpful in alleviating their anxieties. It may provide them with the emotional strength they need to clarify and deal with their feelings.

Olive Flower Essence

Bach olive flower essence is an ideal remedy for women who

are fatigued due to mental and physical exhaustion. This essence is recommended particularly for women who have been trying to conceive for many years, although there is no medical reason for their inability to conceive.

Pine Flower Essence

Those who tend to blame themselves for past mistakes and harbor feelings of failure and lack of accomplishment have found the Bach pine flower essence most helpful. This essence helps people to acknowledge uncomfortable memories of the past without dwelling in them. Pine essence may be helpful for women who may feel a sense of failure and self-blame for their inability to conceive. It may help allow them to come to terms with their feelings and develop a more positive mindset.

She Oak Essence

Made from the female flower of an Australian bush plant, she oak *(Casuarina glauca)* essence has been used by the Aboriginal people of Australia for thousands of years. It is recommended for those who have difficulty conceiving due to emotional blockages caused by feelings of inadequacy or lack of confidence. In addition, women with irregular periods due to hormonal imbalance have found she oak helpful in regulating their cycles and in maintaining healthy cervical mucus.

SUMMING IT UP

Plant oils and essences are holistic healers. For women and men who may have difficulty conceiving due to negative feelings of anxiety, stress, fear, or depression, plant remedies may be helpful. They help to regain the strength and inner balance necessary to heal emotionally, and thus, physically.

Essential oils and flower essences are not to be viewed as

magic bullets. They should be part of a comprehensive wellness program that includes proper diet, adequate exercise, and stress management. Plant remedies, which focus on treating a person's emotional health, can also be combined with the proper herbals, which are significant in promoting good physical health.

8

Alleviating Stress

A relaxed state is believed to help lessen some of the stress that may be linked to infertility, thereby improving chances of conception. In many cases, couples who have trouble conceiving feel frustrated and helpless. They may become anxious, depressed, and even angry. Research has shown that these stress-related feelings may contribute to infertility by causing hormonal imbalances and irregular menstrual cycles in women, and a decrease in sperm production in men. In one study, a number of women who had trouble conceiving for no apparent physical reason, participated in a behavior-modification program. In an effort to reduce their infertility-related stress, they practiced relaxation techniques on a daily basis. Within six months of completing the program, 34 percent of the women became pregnant.

Therapeutic stress-relieving methods, such as meditation, breathing exercises, and muscle relaxation techniques, are excellent for alleviating anxiety, panic, and fear, as well as decreasing chronic tension levels. Massage is also effective for releasing physical tension, restoring energy, and promoting emotional balance. Other benefits of lowered stress levels include a boost in the immune function, an ease in sleep problems, and a reduction in high blood pressure.

RELAXATION TECHNIQUES

The beauty of most relaxation techniques is that they are easy to learn—either by yourself or under the guidance of a professional—and you can perform them at any time. Of course, they won't be able to eliminate all of your stress, but they can help you learn how to relax and bring about a more balanced emotional state.

Also keep in mind that the following relaxation methods, while effective, are not the only ways to cut down on stress. Going on leisurely walks, watching the sun setting at the beach, or chatting on the phone with an old friend can have great calming effects as well. Some people find sitting back and enjoying a great movie to be relaxing. If you find yourself constantly tense and feel the need to unwind, try to create a calming atmosphere whenever possible. Maybe put on some soothing music, dim the lights, and enjoy an occasional glass of wine. Place a few logs in the fireplace and curl up in front of a crackling fire. Soak in a hot bubble bath surrounded by candlelight. The important thing is to use whatever techniques work best for you.

Breathing Exercises

The way you breathe reflects your mood. When you are tense or angry, your breathing tends to become irregular. You gasp when you are surprised, sigh when you are relieved, and probably find it hard to breathe at all when you are frightened. Being able to control your breathing can be a powerful way to gain the upper hand over stress and tension. When your breathing is relaxed, it is difficult to maintain anger or tension.

Try one of the following exercises when you're feeling tense:

CALMING ABDOMINAL BREATHS

*This exercise will help calm jangled nerves
and revitalize the body.*

1. Exhale as completely as you can through your nose.

2. Relax your abdominal muscles and slowly inhale through your nose, sending the air directly to the abdominal area. (This should take anywhere from 5 to 10 seconds.)

3. Purse your lips together and slowly exhale, contracting your abdomen as you exhale and pulling it back toward your spine. (This also should take anywhere from 5 to 10 seconds.)

4. Hold your abdominal muscles in this contracted position for about 5 seconds, and then release.

5. Repeat this exercise at least five times.

QUICK TENSION RELIEVER

This exercise is a quick calmative.

1. Exhale as completely as you can through your nose.

2. Inhale deeply and fully through your nose as you raise your arms upward and reach for the sky. (This should take anywhere from 5 to 10 seconds.)

3. Forcefully exhale as you bend forward at the waist.

4. Inhale again deeply as you straighten up and reach for the sky.

5. Repeat this exercise at least five times.

Muscle Relaxation

People who are constantly under stress carry much of their tension in their muscles. And for most who fall into this category, tense muscles may even appear normal. While performing the following exercise, try to be aware of how much different tense muscles feel from relaxed ones.

MUSCLE RELAXATION EXERCISE

Perform this exercise on a carpeted floor or other soft, padded surface. Wearing comfortable, loose fitting clothing is also recommended but not necessary.

1. Lie on your back.

2. Clench both hands into fists and maintain the tension for 5 seconds. Inhale deeply, then release the tension as you exhale.

3. Bend your arms up, tighten your biceps, and maintain the tension for 5 seconds. Inhale deeply, then release the tension as you exhale.

4. Straighten out your legs, tighten your thigh muscles, and maintain the tension for 5 seconds. Inhale deeply, then release the tension as you exhale.

5. Point your toes down until your shin muscles are taut, and maintain the tension for 5 seconds. Inhale deeply, then release the tension as you exhale.

6. Bend your toes up until your calf muscles are taut, and maintain the tension for 5 seconds. Inhale deeply, then release the tension as you exhale.

7. Pull in your stomach muscles and maintain the tension for 5 seconds. Inhale deeply, then release the tension as you exhale.

8. Squeeze your buttocks together and maintain the tension for 5 seconds. Inhale deeply, then release the tension as you exhale.

9. Bring your shoulders up as close to your ears as possible and maintain the tension for 5 seconds. Inhale deeply, then release the tension as you exhale.

10. Arch your back and maintain the tension for 5 seconds. Inhale deeply, then release the tension as you exhale.

11. Pull your chin down to your chest and maintain the tension for 5 seconds. Inhale deeply, then release the tension as you exhale.

12. Close your eyes tightly, wrinkle your nose, and clench your jaws for 5 seconds. Inhale deeply, then release the tension as you exhale.

Practicing this exercise daily will help you quickly determine which areas of your body are tight. You can then tense and relax the specific areas as needed.

Meditation

Meditation—an activity that calms the mind, keeping it focused and uncluttered—has been practiced for thousands of years. It is a very effective means of treating stress and managing pain. During meditation, the mind is focused on the present, not the past or the future. Most of the hundreds of meditative techniques fall into two main categories: mindfulness and concentrative meditation.

During *mindfulness meditation,* the mind becomes aware of but does not react to its surroundings. While sitting quietly and allowing images of your surroundings to pass through your mind without responding to them, you can achieve a sense of tranquility. To further explain, imagine you are sitting on a lounge chair at the beach. You close your eyes and clear your mind. Suddenly you become aware of sounds—children laughing, a lifeguard's whistle, the crashing of the waves. You notice the heat of the sun on your skin, a trickle of perspiration down your brow, and the sensation of a gentle breeze. You become more and more aware of the sounds, smells, and feelings that surround you, but do not respond to or try to change them. This type of meditation is meant to help you better observe and accept life just as it is, with all of its pleasures, pains, frustrations, and disappointments. It helps you cope better with challenges without becoming emotionally upset by them.

In order to calm the mind when practicing *concentrative meditation*, attention is focused on one's breath, an object, or a repetitive word or phrase. To do this, lie or sit comfortably in a quiet environment with your eyes closed. If you are going to focus on your breath, begin to inhale slowly and deeply through your nose for a count of five, then exhale through your mouth in the same manner. Keeping your mind focused on your breathing rhythm allows your mind to become tranquil.

Be sure to meditate in the proper environment. Choose a quiet place where you will not be disturbed. Although it is not mandatory, playing soft meditational music, which is available in the New Age section of most music stores, is recommended. You might also consider lighting an aromatherapy candle as you meditate. Inhaling the essential oil vapors can greatly enhance relaxation.

Lie or sit comfortably, close your eyes, and try to relax your muscles. As you clear your mind and begin meditating, random thoughts are likely to pop into your head. Try not to focus on these thoughts; simply observe them, then gently return to your focus. Some days you may find yourself distracted continuously as you try to meditate. Again, acknowledge each interruptive thought, then return to your focus. This practice of accepting interruptions is actually a good exercise in developing a tolerant attitude toward the everyday unexpected challenges you face on a daily basis. Try meditating once a day for ten to twenty minutes to reap the greatest benefits.

MASSAGE

Another pleasant, effective way to relax and ease stress and anxiety is through the gentle art of massage. In addition to easing stress, massage, which has been practiced for thousands of years, is used to alleviate pain and heal the body. Although the different therapies that use massage techniques differ slightly, most use finger and full-hand pressure to relax muscles and redistribute energy throughout the body.

Acupressure and reflexology are two popular therapies that utilize massage for treating women with infertility. In a number of cases, women who suffer from endometriosis, habitual miscarriage, fibroid tumors, and amenorrhea have responded well to massage therapy.

Acupressure

In the ancient Chinese healing art of acupressure, finger or thumb pressure is applied to certain points on the body to restore and balance energy, which is known as *chi* (pronounced "chee"). According to Chinese medicine, the body's energy is carried through channels called *meridians.* When these channels become blocked or out of balance, health and well-being are compromised. In acupressure, finger pressure is applied to specific points along the meridians to break down any blockages and regain harmony and balance. Acupressure is actually a noninvasive form of the Chinese practice of acupuncture, in which thin needles are inserted into the same meridian points.

Meridians run along the body, each one corresponding to and named for a different organ. If conception is difficult due to irregular ovulation caused by a hormonal imbalance or, in some instances, fibroid tumors or cystic ovaries, gentle acupressure may be effective. Specific points on the Conception Vessel, Kidney, Spleen, Stomach, and Urinary Bladder meridians are linked to the reproductive system; they are massaged for treating these causes of infertility. Acupressure also can help male infertility caused by a low sperm count, malformed sperm, or poor sperm motility.

According to Elliot Greene, former president of the American Massage Therapy Association, massage can increase the circulation of blood and movement of lymphatic fluids. This encourages the removal of waste and toxins from the body, and improves the transportation of nutrients and oxygen to the cells. Massage can also reduce stress, which can hinder conception.

One of the beauties of acupressure is that it can be performed in the comfort of your own home. It can be self-administered or performed by someone else. Treatments should be given when you are relaxed and comfortable, perhaps after a warm bath just before bedtime. The room should be warm. Before beginning, take a few deep relaxing breaths. You can apply pressure through light clothing or directly to the body.

For the most part, when performing acupressure, you will be using the balls of your thumbs and fingers. Be sure your fingernails are short and smooth so you don't accidentally scratch yourself. Use your fingers and thumb to apply *threshold pressure* to each of the points identified in Figure 8.1 on page 111. Threshold pressure is firm pressure that is just on the verge of becoming painful. Apply from one to three minutes of continuous pressure to each point. Or, you can apply pressure for ten seconds, release for ten seconds, reapply pressure for another ten seconds, release for ten seconds, and repeat the cycle five to ten times. This massage technique can be performed a few times a day. For maximum effects, apply a dab of the Fertility Massage Blend (page 98) or any of the essential oils discussed in Chapter 7 to each area and rub it deeply into each pressure point. (Be sure to blend the essential oil with a carrier oil first.)

Reflexology

Reflexology evolved from an earlier European system called *zone therapy,* which was introduced in the United States by laryngologist William Fitzgerald, M.D. It uses therapeutic pressure on specific reflex areas located on the feet, which correspond to internal glands and organs. Stimulating the

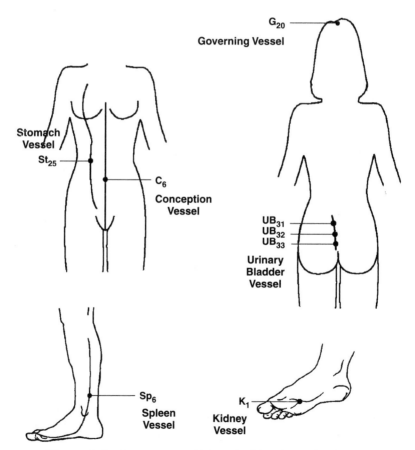

Figure 8.1. Acupressure Points for Treating Infertility

proper reflex area has a direct effect on the associated body part. It allows the energy to flow freely along the meridian, and the part of the body associated with that reflex point can once again function properly.

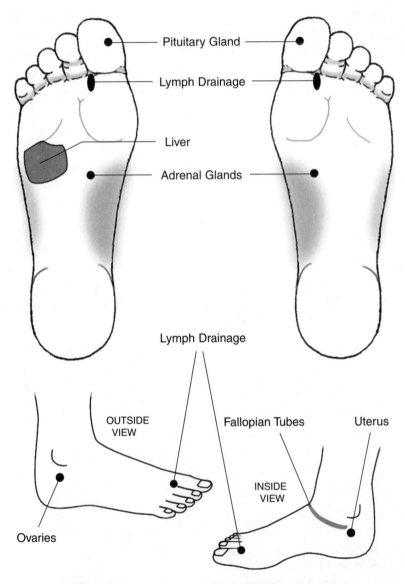

Figure 8.2. Reflex Areas for Treating Infertility

In addition to revitalizing energy flow, improving circulation, and ridding the body of toxins, reflexology also helps relieve pain, reduce stress, and promote general balance and harmony. Also, this form of massage may help regulate hormone levels, which, in turn, can stabilize irregular menstrual cycles, encouraging ovulation. It may also be helpful for women with fibroid tumors and endometriosis.

Although reflex areas in the hands are not as sensitive as those in the feet, they can be massaged if there is an injury to the foot. Be aware that reflexology should not be performed on those with severe foot problems, osteoporosis, or infections. During self-treatment, if the foot area cannot be reached, specific areas of the hand can be massaged instead.

Before self treatment, it is recommended to pay a visit to a reflexologist, who will show you the effective massage techniques. Once you have determined the proper reflex areas and know the correct massage methods, either you or a partner can stimulate the proper reflex points. Figure 8.2 points out the reflex areas of the foot that are massaged to encourage fertility. Massaging each point up to three minutes, three times a day.

SUMMING IT UP

Stress is one of the underlying factors in a number of health-related conditions, including infertility. Practicing relaxation techniques can help reduce stress and encourage conception. As you have seen in this chapter, there are a number of techniques—deep breathing and muscle exercises, meditation, massage, and activities as simple as daily walks—that can help you control the stress in your life and increase your odds of conception.

A Final Word

Infertility can be the result of a number of causes. In some instances, such as those resulting from tubal, ovarian, or uterine conditions, surgery or other technological procedures may be helpful. However, in certain cases, couples fail to conceive for reasons that are not always apparent. Unlikely factors, such as stress, vitamin deficiency, and exposure to environmental toxins, can be some of the factors behind hormone imbalance or other subtle causes that impede conception.

Incorporating a holistic approach to health—one in which the mind as well as the body is kept strong and well-balanced—has been the key for many couples in increasing their odds of conceiving. And in most instances, it takes only a few simple lifestyle adjustments. For instance, eliminating tension and anxiety from your life by employing stress management techniques, as well as getting proper nutrition from foods and dietary supplements, can help promote internal balance and strengthen the reproductive systems of both women and men. Using certain homeopathic remedies and essential oils from plants and flowers also have been effective in encouraging a sound, healthy mind and body.

I began taking fertility drugs to help rebalance my reproductive hormones, but their side effects—hot flashes, strong mood swings, and migraine headaches—prompted me to seek out gentler, more natural methods of encouraging conception. I found a doctor who was qualified in the field of complementary medicine. After undergoing a thorough physical examination, he introduced me to a number of natural methods for overcoming infertility. While I was under his care, he kept a close watch on my uneven hormone levels, which had been the source of my inability to conceive.

In addition to the advice and guidance of my physician, I frequently used my intuition, my "gut feeling," to select the types of treatment with which I felt most comfortable. Do not be afraid to listen to what your heart and mind tell you. I believe a modicum of intuition, professional guidance, and inner focus will help give you the strength to choose a course of action that is right for you.

Obviously, there is no panacea for infertility, and dealing with it can be difficult and frustrating. However, there is reason to be hopeful. In many cases, the strength of treating this condition lies in the ability to enhance overall health by healing the body-mind state. I found that a diet rich in fresh vegetables and whole grains, combined with regular exercise, vitamin and herbal supplements, and a stress-free environment helped my body obtain the inner balance it needed to facilitate conception. The knowledge I have gained in my quest to become pregnant is presented in this book, in the hope that it will help do the same for you.

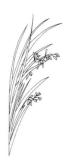

Bibliography

Alternative Medicine. Compiled by the Burton Goldberg Group. Puyallup, WA: Future Medicine Publishing, 1993.

Balch, James F., and Phyllis A. Balch. *Prescription for Nutritional Healing,* 2nd edition. Garden City Park, NY: Avery Publishing Group, 1997.

Balch, Phyllis A., and James F. Balch. *Prescription for Dietary Wellness.* Greenfield, IN: PAB Books, 1992.

Beal, MW. "Acupuncture and acupressure. Applications to women's reproductive health care." *Journal Nurse Midwifery,* 44.3: 217–230, May–June, 1999.

Brown, Donald J. *Herbal Prescriptions for Better Health.* Rocklin, CA: Prima Publishing, 1995.

Clubb, Elizabeth, and Jane Knight. *Fertility.* Brunel House, UK: David & Charles, 1996.

Cooke, Cynthia W., and Susan Dworkin. *The Ms. Guide to a Woman's Health.* Garden City, NY: Doubleday & Company, 1979.

Cramer, DW, H. Xu, and T. Sahi. "Adult hypolactasia, milk consumption, and age-specific fertility." *American Journal of Epidemiology,* 139.3: 282–289, 1994.

Dawson, EB, WA Harris, MC Teter, and LC Powell. "Effect of ascorbic acid supplementation on the sperm quality of smokers." *Fertility and Sterility,* 58.5: 1034–1039, 1992.

Domar, A., M. Seibel, and H. Benson. "The mind/body program for infertility: a new behavioural treatment approach for women with infertility." *Fertility and Sterility,* 53.2: 246–249, 1990.

Franklin, Robert R., and Dorothy Ray Breckman. *In Pursuit of Fertility.* New York: Henry Holt & Company, 1990.

Gay, Kathlyn. *Silent Killers.* New York: Impact Books, 1988.

Geva, E., B. Bartov, N. Zabludovsky, et al. "The effect of antioxidant treatment on human spermatozoa and fertilization rate in an in vitro fertilization program." *Fertility and Sterility,* 66.3: 430–434, 1996.

Gottlieb, Bill. *New Choices in Natural Healing*. Emmaus, PA: Rodale Press, 1995.

Green, BB., et al. "Risk of ovulatory infertility in relation to body weight." *Fertility and Sterility*, 50.9: 621–626, 1988.

Gursche, Siegfried. *Encyclopedia of Natural Healing*. Burnaby, BC, Canada: Alive Books, 1997.

Harvey, Clare G., and Amanda Cochrane. *The Encyclopedia of Flower Remedies*. San Francisco, CA: Thorsons, 1995.

Hoffman, David. *An Elder's Herbal*. Rochester, VT: Healing Arts Press, 1993.

Howard, JM., S. Davies, and A. Hunnisett. "Red cell magnesium and glutathione peroxidase in infertile women, effects of oral supplementation with magnesium and selenium." *Magnesium Research*, 7.1: 49–57, March 1994.

Hughes, CL, Jr. "Phytochemical mimicry of reproductive hormones and modulation of herbivore fertility by phytoestrogens." *Environmental Health Perspectives*, 78: 171–175, 1988.

Joesoef, MR., V. Beral, SO Aral, RT Rolfs, and DW Cramer. "Fertility and use of cigarettes, alcohol, marijuana, and cocaine." *Annals of Epidemiology*, 3(6): 592–594, November 1993.

Lark, Susan. *Fibroid Tumors and Endometriosis: A Self-Help Book*. Berkeley, CA: Celestial Arts, 1995.

Sanyal, SN. "Ten Years of Research on an Oral Contraceptive from Pisum Sativum." *Science and Culture*, 25.12: 661–665, 1960.

Scott, Julian, and Susan Scott. *Natural Medicine for Women*. New York: Avon Books, 1991.

Sobel, David S., and Robert Ornstein. *The Healthy Mind Healthy Body Handbook*. New York: Patient Education Media, Inc., 1996.

Teeguarden, Ron. *Chinese Tonic Herbs*. New York: Japan Publications, 1984.

Terhune, Mary. *Fertile Ground Network*. http://www.tiac.net/ users/ fertile, November 1, 1996.

Wasser, SK. "Reproductive control in wild baboons measured by fecal steroids." *Biology of Reproduction*, 55(2): 393–399, 1996.

Wilcox, A., et al. "Caffeinated beverages and decreased fertility." *Lancet*, 2: 1473–1476, 1988.

Wilson, Roberta. *Aromatherapy*. Garden City Park, NY: Avery Publishing Group, 1994.

Worwood, Valerie Ann. *The Fragrant Pharmacy: A Complete Guide to Aromatherapy & Essential Oils*. London, UK: Bantam Books, 1991.

Zand, Janet, Alan N. Spreen, and James B. LaValle. *Smart Medicine for Healthier Living*. Garden City Park, NY: Avery Publishing Group, 1999.

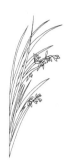

Index